# Surgery of the Pancreas and Spleen

W0036731

Kirby I. Bland • Michael G. Sarr
Markus W. Büchler • Attila Csendes
Oliver James Garden • John Wong
(Editors)

# Surgery of the Pancreas and Spleen

Handbooks in General Surgery

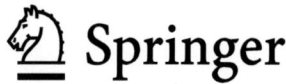 Springer

*Editors*

Kirby I. Bland
University of Alabama
Birmingham
Department of Surgery
Birmingham Alabama
USA

Attila Csendes
University of Chile
Clinical Hospital
Department of Surgery
Santiago
Chile

Michael G. Sarr
Mayo Clinic
Division of Gastroenterologic &
General Surgery
Rochester Minnesota
USA

Oliver James Garden
University of Edinburgh
Royal Infirmary
Department of Surgery
Edinburgh
United Kingdom

Markus W. Büchler
Universitätsklinikum Heidelberg
Chirurgische Klinik
Abt. Allgemeine, Viszerale und
Unfallchirurgie
Heidelberg
Germany

John Wong
Queen Mary Hospital
Department of Surgery
Hong Kong

ISBN 978-1-84996-368-8        e-ISBN 978-1-84996-369-5
DOI 10.1007/978-1-84996-369-5
Springer London Dordrecht Heidelberg New York

British Library Cataloguing in Publication Data
A catalogue record for this book is available from the British Library

Library of Congress Control Number: 2011921907

© Springer-Verlag London Limited 2011
First published in 2009 as part of Operational Risk: Practice and Implementation, edited by Kathryn E. Dinan, Markus W. Blochwitz, Anita Cramer
© Nestor-Flacher, Michael C. Sara & John Wang, ISBN 978-1-84628-873-6
Whilst we have made considerable efforts to contact all holders of copyright material contained in this book, we may have failed to locate some of them. Should holders wish to contact the Publisher, we will be happy to come to some arrangement with them.
Apart from any fair dealing for the purposes of research or private study, or criticism or review, as permitted under the Copyright, Designs and Patents Act 1988, this publication may only be reproduced, stored or transmitted, in any form or by any means, with the prior permission in writing of the publishers, or in the case of reprographic reproduction in accordance with the terms of licences issued by the Copyright Licensing Agency. Enquiries concerning reproduction outside those terms should be sent to the publishers.
The use of registered names, trademarks, etc. in this publication does not imply, even in the absence of a specific statement, that such names are exempt from the relevant laws and regulations and therefore free for general use.
The publisher makes no representation, express or implied, with regard to the accuracy of the information contained in this book and cannot accept any legal responsibility or liability for any errors or omissions that may be made.

Cover design: eStudio Calamar, Figueres/Berlin

Printed on acid-free paper

Springer is part of Springer Science+Business Media (www.springer.com)

ISBN  978-1-84996-368-8          e-ISBN  978-1-84996-369-5
DOI  10.1007/978-1-84996-369-5
Springer London Dordrecht Heidelberg New York

British Library Cataloguing in Publication Data
A catalogue record for this book is available from the British Library

Library of Congress Control Number: 2010937967

*Cover design*: eStudioCalamar, Figueres/Berlin

Printed on acid-free paper

Springer is part of Springer Science+Business Media (www.springer.com)

# Preface

The editors designed the original textbook, *General Surgery: Principles and International Practice,* from which this shorter paperback monograph on surgery of the pancreas and spleen was taken to be an accessible, concise, and state-of-the-art volume that explores and documents evolutionary principles in the practice of surgery. This work is aimed at the general surgeon and the resident in training. The scientific community continues to witness extraordinary advances in the therapy of both benign and malignant surgical diseases of various organ sites. Much of this progress has been evident over the past decade with new concepts and techniques of management that allow the surgeon to integrate this discipline with medicine, pharmacology, immunology, biostatistics, pathology, genetics, medical and radiation oncology, and diagnostic radiology and imaging. Further, each of these major disciplines contributes a small component for the diagnostic and therapeutic approaches to clinical care; hence the comprehensive planning, integration, and provision of patient care throughout the preoperative, intraoperative, and postoperative phases of care remains essential in the successful practice of our specialty.

The editors acknowledge that the aim of this work is to provide an illustrative, instructive, and comprehensive review that depicts the rationale of basic operative principles essential to surgical therapy. In organizing this monograph, the editors chose authors renowned in the disciplines for illustrating, forming, and depicting in a comprehensive fashion the surgical therapy expectant for metabolic, infectious, endocrine, and neoplastic abnormalities in adult and pediatric patients **from a truly international and multi-continental perspective.** The editors and authors were chosen carefully from across geographies and also from multi-cultural and diverse locations. While the authors consider this text to be inclusive regarding the technical and operative conditions for perioperative care in this field, its purpose should not be intended to replace standard textbooks of surgery nor should it be considered complete in its coverage of pathophysiologic disorders. In contrast, this monograph is organized to familiarize practicing surgeons, residents, and fellows with state-of-the-art surgical principles and techniques essential to contemporary practice. Therefore, the tenor of this monograph on surgery of the pancreas and spleen has been developed to coexist with other major surgical reference texts that are dedicated—some in more comprehensive fashion—to the therapy of individual organs of systemic diseases. This monograph is much more a "working text" for the practicing surgeon with emphasis on diagnosis and treatment of pancreatic and splenic disorders. Along with this monograph, nine other paperback monographs are available and focus on the general principles of surgery, trauma, critical care, esophagus and stomach, small bowel, colorectal, liver and biliary, oncology, and endocrine organs, all adapted from the primary textbook—*General Surgery: Principles and International Practice.*

The chapters in this monograph on surgery of the pancreas and spleen include a condensed bibliography of highly selective journal articles, reviews, and text. In this manner of attempting to be concise, we hope to provide a precise focus for the education of the reader relative to accepted surgical principles involved in patient care. Moreover, the editors have sought to provide a counterpoint view for the selection of therapy by presenting at the opening of each chapter a list of "Pearls and Pitfalls" that highlight particular concerns or controversies. The chapters provide pertinent, though not exhaustive, summaries of anatomy and physiology, a history of surgical illness, and stages of operative approaches with relevant technical considerations outlined in an easily under-standable manner. Complications are reviewed when appro-priate for the organ system, diseases, and problem. The text is supported amply by line drawings and photographs that depict anatomic or technical principles. The editors have made every attempt to minimize duplicative or repetitive discussions except when controversial or state-of-the-art issues are presented. Moreover, the editors have attempted to ensure that accurate presentations and illustrations depict properly the most complex problems confronted by the gen-eral surgeon.

Finally, in an attempt to address advances in contemporary concepts, the text has been organized to address in detail expeditious, safe, and anatomically accurate operations and incorporate standard as well as evolving surgical principles and techniques. These principles have been tested in the clin-ics of valid scientific knowledge and are well supported by the time-tested approaches that have been provided by prac-ticing surgeons. The editors are excited to be able to respond to the challenge of developing a truly international text and are indeed hopeful that our readers will find this focused monograph on surgery of the pancreas and spleen to be a repository of insight, useful, and timely information.

Kirby I. Bland
Michael G. Sarr
Markus W. Büchler
Attila Csendes
O. James Garden
John Wong

# Contents

# Contributors

**Åke Andrén-Sandberg, MD, PhD**
Professor of Surgery, Department of Surgery, Karolinska
University Hospital at Huddinge, Stockholm, Sweden

**Markus W. Büchler, MD**
Professor of Surgery and Chairman, Department of General
and Visceral Surgery, University of Heidelberg, Heidelberg,
Germany

**Patricio Burdiles, MD, FACS**
Chief, Digestive Surgical Unit, Department of Surgery,
Clinical Hospital University of Chile Santiago, Chile

**Juan Luis Calisto, MD**
Department of Laparoscopic Surgery, Clinica Anglo
Americana, Lima, Peru

**Miguel Caracoche, MD**
Department of Surgery, Hospital de Clínicas "José de San
Martín," Universidad de Buenos Aires, Buenos Aires,
Argentina

**Ross Carter, MBChB, MD, FRCS**
Consultant, General Surgeon, Department of Surgery,
Glasgow Royal Infirmary, Glasgow, UK

**José Eduardo M. Cunha, MD**
Department of Gastroenterology, São Paulo University
School of Medicine, São Paulo, Brazil

**Luis A. Durand, MD**
Department of Internal Medicine, Hospital de Clínicas "José de San Martín", Universidad de Buenos Aires, Argentina

**Douglas B. Evans, MD**
Professor of Surgery, Department of Surgery, University of Texas M D Anderson Cancer Center, Houston, TX, USA

**Pedro Ferraina, MD, PhD, FACS**
Professor and Chairman, Department of Surgery, Hospital de Clínicas "José de San Martín," Universidad de Buenos Aires, Buenos Aires, Argentina

**Ariel Ferraro, MD**
Department of Surgery, Hospital de Clínicas "José de San Martín," Universidad de Buenos Aires, Buenos Aires, Argentina

**José Jukemura, MD**
Department of Biliary & Pancreatic Surgery, Faculty of Medicine, University of São Paulo, São Paulo, Brazil

**Debra L. Kennamer, MD**
Professor, Department of Anesthesiology and Pain Medicine, University of Texas M D Anderson Cancer Center, Houston, TX, USA

**Yaira Lopez, MD**
Resident, Digestive Surgery, Department of Surgery, Clinical Hospital University of Chile Santiago, Chile

**Marcel C. C. Machado, MD, FACS**
Professor, Department of Surgery, University of São Paulo, São Paulo, Brazil

**Colin J. McKay, MBChB, MD, FRCS**
Senior Lecturer, Department of Surgery, Glasgow Royal Infirmary, Glasgow, UK

**Melinda M. Mortenson, MD**
Surgical Oncology Fellow, Department of Surgical
Oncology, University of Texas M D Anderson Cancer
Center, Houston, TX, USA

**Mario S. Nahmod, MD**
Department of Surgery, Hospital de Clínicas "José de San
Martín," Universidad de Buenos Aires, Buenos Aires,
Argentina

**Robert T.A. Padbury, MBBS FRACS PhD**
Director, Division of Surgical and Specialty Services,
Flinders Medical Centre, Bedford Park, Australia

**Martín Palavecino, MD**
Fellow, HPB Surgery and Liver Transplantation, General
Surgery Service, Hospital Italiano de Buenos Aires, Buenos
Aires, Argentina

**Juan Pekolj, MD, PhD, FACS**
Chief of HPB, Surgery Section, General Surgery Service,
Hospital Italiano de Buenos Aires, Buenos Aires, Argentina

**Luis Poggi, MD, FACS**
Department of Laparoscopic Surgery, Clinica Anglo
Americana, Lima, Peru

**Richard A. Prinz, MD, FACS**
Professor and Chairman, Department of General Surgery,
Rush Medical College, Chicago, IL, USA

**George H. Sakorafas, MD, PhD**
Surgeon and Lecturer, 4th Department of Surgery, Athens
University Medical School, Athens, Greece

**Michael G. Sarr, MD**
James C. Mason Professor of Surgery, Department of Surgery,
Mayo Clinic College of Medicine, Rochester, MN, USA

**Carmen C. Solórzano, MD, FACS**
Associate Professor of Surgery, Department of Surgery,
Rush Medical College, Chicago, IL, USA

**Eric P. Tamm, MD**
Associate Professor, Department of Diagnostic Radiology,
University of Texas M D Anderson Cancer Center, Houston,
TX, USA

**Huamin Wang, MD, PhD**
Assistant Professor, Department of Pathology, University of
Texas M D Anderson Cancer Center, Houston, TX, USA

**Andrew L. Warshaw, MD**
W. Gerald Austen Professor and Chair, Department of
Surgery, Massachusetts General Hospital, Boston, MA, USA

**Jens Werner, MD**
Professor of Surgery, Department of General and Visceral
Surgery, University of Heidelberg, Heidelberg, Germany

# Part I
# Pancreas — Benign

# 1
# Management of Necrotizing Pancreatis

**Ross Carter and Colin J. McKay**

## Pearls and Pitfalls

- The management of necrotizing pancreatitis has changed dramatically in the last 10 years.
- Open operative necrosectomy has given way to multi-modal focused interventional techniques.
- Early management involves critical care principles, nutritional support, and selective use of endoscopic retrograde cholangiography/sphincterotomy and antibiotics.
- Not all patients with infected necrosis will require intervention; also the goal is to delay the need for intervention for 4–12 weeks when the necrosis has become walled off.
- Infected areas can be approached percutaneously via a combined radiologic/nephroscopic drainage, laparoscopically via a transgastric approach, or endoscopically via a transgastric approach – all are potentially complementary.
- Even the patient with infected necrosis with not-yet-walled-off necrosis may benefit by percutaneous radiologic/nephroscopic drainage.

Bleeding complicating the management of necrotizing pancreatitis is best managed by angiography and transvascular embolization.

K.I. Bland et al. (eds.), *Surgery of the Pancreas and Spleen*, DOI: 10.1007/978-1-84996-369-5_1,
© Springer-Verlag London Limited 2011

# Introduction

Approximately 15% of patients with acute pancreatitis will have evidence of hypoperfusion of the pancreas on a contrast-enhanced computed tomography of the abdomen. The necrotic process usually is not limited to the pancreas, and peri-pancreatic necrosis may occur alongside relatively minor degrees of parenchymal damage (Fig. 1.1). After initiation of an acute attack of pancreatitis, the pancreatic and peri-pancreatic necrotizing process extends over the next 48 h, associated with interstitial edema. The edema within this essentially solid, inflammatory mass coalesces subsequently into acute fluid collections containing a variable amount of devitalized tissue. With maturity, the demarcation between viable and necrotic tissue becomes established, and the collection becomes lined with granulation tissue. Control of the necrosis and prevention of infection within that necrosis have been assumed in the past to be the key to clinical resolution, leading to a proactive approach toward identification and early intervention for secondary infection of pancreatic

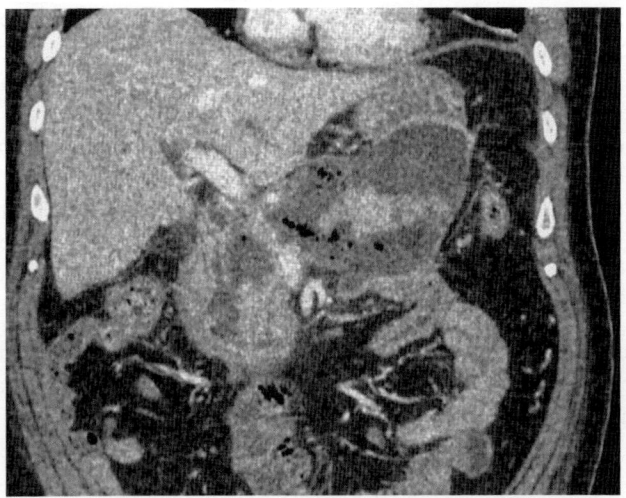

FIGURE 1.1. Infected pancreatic and peri-pancreatic necrosis.

necrosis. In recent years, it has become clear that, while there is undoubtedly a relationship between the extent of necrosis, infection and outcome, survival is related more intimately to the presence of systemic organ failure.

Indeed, marked necrosis and occasionally infection within the necrosis can occur without substantive systemic upset, and fatal multiple organ failure can occur without substantial pancreatic necrosis.

In managing patients with severe acute pancreatitis, there are two distinct phases during which intervention is considered: *Early* (within 1–2 weeks of admission), where the main concern is minimizing the mortality from multiple organ dysfunction syndrome (MODS), and *late* (from 2 weeks onward), during which septic complications, particularly infected pancreatic necrosis (IPN), are the primary concern, whether or not MODS is present.

# Early Management

The dynamic pattern of organ dysfunction within the early phase of the inflammatory process dictates appropriate management primarily through respiratory and circulatory support. There is no role for operative intervention, except in the occasional patient with hemorrhagic complications or visceral perforation. Approximately 40% of deaths in acute pancreatitis occur within the first week of illness, many of these occurring within 72 h. The management of patients with severe early MODS remains one of the most challenging aspects in the management of acute pancreatitis. Specific therapy with somatostatin or its analogues or antiproteases have not proven to be helpful in large clinical trials, nor has the cytokine antagonist lexipafant, despite promising results in early studies. Early recognition and management of MODS in an appropriate intensive care environment is the mainstay of management, but several areas with specific interventions should be considered:

1. CT: Patients with deteriorating MODS within 48h of admission have an anticipated mortality of approximately 50%.

An abdominal CT maybe considered to confirm the suspected diagnosis, and in particular to exclude perforated viscus. Knowledge that a patient with early MODS has extensive pancreatic necrosis does not change management at this stage.

2. Endoscopic retrograde cholangiography(ERC): One of the difficult decisions faced by clinicians is when to undertake ERC in a patient with acute pancreatitis who is deteriorating clinically. Published evidence is conflicting and much is said on the subject that cannot be justified by an objective appraisal of the evidence. In practice, emergency ERC in a patient on the brink of requiring assisted ventilation is not without risk. On the basis of results from the largest randomized trial, we have abandoned urgent ERC in acute pancreatitis, except for the clear indication of actual or suspected cholangitis or worsening jaundice. The coexistence of acute pancreatitis and cholangitis does need to be considered however, and a jaundiced patient with evidence of systemic inflammatory response syndrome (SIRS) will, in our institution, undergo urgent ERC with endoscopic sphincterotomy.

3. Prophylactic antibiotics: Contradictory results from clinical trials with widely varying antibiotic protocols have led to persistent controversy over the role for prophylactic antibiotics in patients with pancreatic necrosis. In practice however, many patients are begun on antibiotics by referring institutions or by the local medical teams. Our own preference is to withhold antibiotics, except for culture-proven sepsis, but if antibiotics are commenced, we continue their use for a defined course of 7–10 days. Every attempt is made to avoid the situation of patients receiving repeated courses of different antibiotics on the basis of continuing pyrexia (an expected manifestation of SIRS in severe pancreatitis) but in the absence of proven infection, because this practice runs the risk of selecting out hospital-acquired organisms and developing septic complications with these resistant organisms or fungi.

4. Enteral nutrition: Patients with multiple organ dysfunction
   syndrome (MODS) and pancreatic necrosis can be expected
   to have a protracted, difficult illness with profound weight
   loss as a common feature. Nutritional support will not prevent this weight loss but is an essential component of the
   multidisciplinary management of these patients to minimize
   infections and metabolic complications. Total parenteral
   nutrition was favored formerly, in the assumption that pancreatic "rest" was important for recovery; however, randomized trials have shown the safety of enteral nutrition, and, as
   in other critical illness, the enteral route of delivery is increasingly favored. In our institution, nasogastric feeding is used
   when tolerated, but many patients require placement of a
   nasojejunal tube due to gastric stasis. Occasionally, patients
   have difficulty with gastrointestinal absorption of the tube-
   feeding formulas, and if this persists despite use of predi-
   gested "elemental" formulas, then combined feeding with
   parenteral nutrition and low volume enteral feed maybe
   required. There is no evidence that early enteral nutrition
   itself influences the outcome from acute pancreatitis.

## Management of Late Complications

It was assumed previously that all patients in whom bacterial
(or fungal) colonization of the devitalized pancreatic/peri-
pancreatic tissue occurred required intervention, and that the
patient would not recover until complete necrosectomy/
debridement had been achieved. Also, operative intervention
in patients with established MODS but in the absence of
infection was associated with a very poor outcome, leading to
attempts at early confirmation of infection by CT-guided, fine
needle aspiration (FNA), with a view to operative intervention before secondary MODS developed. Not all patients
with infected necrosis, however, are unwell, and, consequently, the universal requirement for eventual intervention
is overstated. In most surgical conditions, sepsis-driven
MODS results from inadequate drainage of the septic focus.

Within the Glasgow Unit, our approach has evolved to one of sepsis control rather than radical debridement of necrosis.

There has also been a tendency for specialist centers to manage all patients by way of a single treatment approach, despite a wide range of presentations. We contend that an armamentarium of different approaches might be appropriate depending on the anatomic location of the collection, the duration from presentation, the presence of co-morbidities, and the extent of MODS. Several techniques may be employed over the duration of treatment in any single patient, and each technique should be seen as complementary rather than exclusive.

In general our approach is to avoid intervention unless we suspect that the patient's clinical condition is being compromised by an un-drained, presumably infected collection. The initiator for sequential imaging, usually by way of CT, is, therefore, a secondary deterioration in organ failure scores or serial biochemistry, rather than routine interval CT imaging or a protocol-driven repetitive FNA approach. In those patients in whom clinical sepsis is suspected, contrast enhanced CT is performed with a view to probable intervention, the nature of which is determined by the clinical condition of the patient and the time course from initial presentation.

## Clinical Pathology of Late Collections in Acute Pancreatitis

The approach to the management of a deteriorating patient with a pancreatic/peri-pancreatic collection is determined by the time course from presentation and the clinical condition of the patient. An over-aggressive approach in a patient with established MODS can lead to further de-compensation and often death. The process of maturation, and "walling off" of the necrosis with separation and partial liquefaction of the solid components within a collection, takes up to 12 weeks to complete, during which several stages can be recognized, and the clinico-radiologic balance will determine the optimum intervention.

1. True pancreatic necrosis

There are two peaks in the mortality associated with acute pancreatitis. The majority of late deaths occur in the group that develops sepsis-driven complications relatively early (2–4 weeks), when organization of the peri-pancreatic collection is incomplete and the ability of radiologic means of effective intervention is limited. It is in these patients that MODS is common, and in the critically ill, a staged approach with initial radiologic drainage to downstage and control the septic process, followed by definitive management during a therapeutic window of improvement, may be appropriate.

Aggressive, open operative exploration encounters semi-adherent devitalized tissue which, if removed, results in bleeding. Staged open approaches of open laparostomy, closed packing, or closed lavage are all attempts at controlling the pancreatic and peri-pancreatic sepsis in the presence of incomplete debridement. For some time, we have argued that complete debridement is unnecessary, and, provided adequate control of sepsis can be maintained, organ failure will recover, allowing removal of necrosis to be achieved in a delayed fashion.

It is in these patients that we most commonly utilize the percutaneous necrosectomy approach, the aim of the procedure being to control the sepsis rather than to achieve complete debridement. Within 24–36 h of the initial CT-guided puncture and drainage of the area of infection, the tract of the drainage catheter is dilated, the cavity is irrigated under vision, and a larger drainage catheter is inserted. Under general anesthesia, the patient is placed supine with sand-bags used to optimize access to the drain site, ideally a left flank approach via the lieno-colic window; this approach provides direct access to the pancreatic bed and promotes dependent drainage. Using a Seldinger approach, a guide wire is used to exchange the drainfora30FG balloon dilator (COOK Limited, Herts, UK) followed by a graduated dilator to 34FG to allow insertion of an Amplatz sheath. Using a modified nephrostomy, rigid-rod lens system, cavity lavage is initiated using warmed saline infused via a rapid infuser until the fluid within the cavity allows adequate visualization. At the initial procedure, the aim is to achieve adequate and sustainable sepsis control, rather than complete debridement, and so, while piecemeal removal of loose necrotic material is performed, prolonged attempts at debridement during the initial procedure are avoided, because these maneuvers may result in worsening sepsis and systemic compromise. An 8 Fr umbilical catheter is sutured to a 32 Fr PORTEX chest drain (SIMS Portex Limited, Kent, UK) in two positions, and this catheter assembly is advanced into the cavity. A continuous, postoperative closed lavage at 250 ml/h is begun and continued postoperatively. A median of three secondary interval procedures are usually required over the coming weeks, hopefully in a patient with improving organ dysfunction and controlled sepsis.

## 2. Walled-off pancreatic necrosis (WOPN)

In general, patients with walled-off necrosis are in reasonable health, having been nursed through the initial 4–12 weeks of the illness (Fig. 1.2). Pressure symptoms, pain, inability to eat, non-resolution of a large collection/abdominal mass, or occasionally infection are the common indications for intervention. Previous reports recommending intervention for non-resolving collections before this time have little clinical basis. Significant organ dysfunction or sepsis is rare, and our approach is based on managing the collection as a single intervention. Our preference is for a transgastric gastrocystostomy approach allowing adequate drainage and removal of any separated necrotic material at the same time. This procedure maybe performed either by an open operation or by a laparoscopic, intra-visceral approach. Both approaches have the advantage that a simultaneous cholecystectomy (with cholangiogram) can be performed. The open approach has been described extensively. The laparoscopic approach involves insertion of an infra-umbilical blunt port using a Hasson technique.

Because intra-abdominal inflammatory adhesions are common, a Veress needle approach is not recommended. An

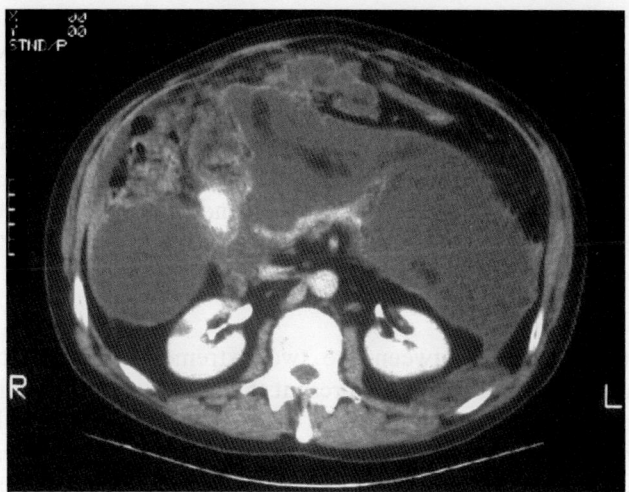

FIGURE 1.2. Walled-off pancreatic necrosis.

endoscope is passed perorally, and 100 ml of saline is instilled into the duodenum to act as a sump. The stomach is inflated using the endoscope, and through use of dual imaging (endo-gastric and intraperitoneal), 3 "Step ports" (Tyco Healthcare Limited, Hampshire, UK) (2 × 12 mm and1 × 5 mm) are then inserted through the abdominal wall and into the stomach. These tracks are then dilated to allow insertion of the laparo-scope intragastrically via the transabdominal approach. The WOPN is identified on laparoscopic Ultrasonography after diathermy-assisted puncture of the cavity. A gastrocystos-tomy (10–12 cm length) is then created using three firings of the Endo GIA stapler. Any necrosis can be removed and placed in the stomach. The ports are removed, and the gastro-tomy puncture sites are closed by intracorporeal suture. An endoscopic technique has been described as well.

In some patients, large areas of WOPN require drainage, but the patients are either frail, morbidly obese, or serious co-morbidity makes an operative approach unattractive. In these patients, we utilize an aggressive, EUS-guided endoscopic gastrocystotomy approach. EUS-guided gastrocystotomy is modified to allow dilatation of the gastrocystotomy tract using a 15 mm balloon at the time of initial puncture. Two double pigtail stents maintain tract patency in addition to cavity lavage using a nasocystic catheter, irrigating the cavity using warmed dialysis fluid at 100 ml/h. Secondary endoscopic procedures to allow tract dilatation (15 mm), occasionally combined with intracavity endoscopy and piecemeal debridement, are usually required prior to resolution.

## 3. Intermediate

Patients falling between the two extremes of pancreatic necrosis and WOPN often present the greatest management challenge. Timing and choice of intervention can be difficult, and the wrong choice has the potential to worsen the clinical situation. Between 3 and 10 weeks after onset of the pancreatitis, patients with infected pancreatic necrosis maybe managed by a variety of approaches. In those patients with ongoing MODS, our approach is similar to that in patients with early IPN, with percutaneous drainage and necrosectomy. Patients with no organ dysfunction but demonstrable infected necrosis maybe managed by laparoscopic transgastric drainage if sufficiently late in the course of the illness, but this technique is less suitable for patients less than 8–10 weeks from onset. In this situation, we consider giving antibiotics and trying to delay intervention. We have observed complete resolution of the infected area in some patients in this group with antibiotic therapy alone, but in most cases, laparoscopic or endoscopic drainage will prove to be necessary. Patients showing signs of clinical deterioration while on antibiotic therapy will undergo percutaneous necrosectomy if less than 8 weeks from illness onset.

A percutaneous necrosectomy approach will result in a prolonged hospital stay, and inevitably serial interventions compared to a single transgastric intervention. Our general aim, therefore, is to manage these patients with the algorithm addressing management of WOPN, reserving a percutaneous approach for those with marked co-morbidity or organ dysfunction.

### 4. Pseudocyst

By definition, a "pseudocyst" contains minimal necrosis; the management of pseudocysts, whether infected or not, in patients after an attack of acute pancreatitis, is usually by trans-gastric drainage. After acute pancreatitis, many patients with apparent pseudocysts will have marked necrosis which may not be obvious on CT but which is identified easily on MRI or at EUS. Transpapillary drainage, as favored for simple pseudocysts, runs the risk of infecting these necrotic collections, and therefore we favor transgastric drainage under EUS guidance. Where there is minimal necrosis and no infection, two pigtail stents are left in place without the need for a naso-cyst lavage catheter; in contrast, when there is significant necrosis, these patients are managed for WOPN by post-procedural lavage. Follow-up transabdominal ultrasonography is carried out within 48 h to ensure that the cyst has been drained adequately, and if not, further endoscopic dilatation of the gastrocystostomy track is carried out.

Rarely, patients may have persistent pseudocysts despite endoscopic drainage; this situation is usually related to a "disconnected duct syndrome" which occurs when central pancreatic necrosis results in disconnection of the duct in the pancreatic tail with the proximal pancreatic duct. These patients usually need a distal pancreatectomy, although in patients with serious mitigating co-morbidity, prolonged relief can be obtained by EUS-guided drainage, leaving the stents in situ for an indefinite period.

# Management of Other Complications in Patients with Infected Pancreatic Necrosis

### 1. Bleeding

Bleeding into the retroperitoneum is evident from the presence of fresh blood in a lavage catheter. Gastrointestinal bleeding may also occur, but most bleeding is associated with a retroperitoneal source with fistulation into the GI tract.

In either situation, the preferred management is mesenteric angiography and embolization. The usual bleeding site is the splenic artery or less commonly, the gastroduodenal artery, but other sites may be involved, particularly where there is extensive necrosis of the pancreatic head. A small "herald" bleed is common, and ward staff must be alert to this complication so that urgent arrangements for angiography are made before the inevitable massive bleeding ensues. Failure of mesenteric embolization necessitates operative intervention, but in these cases, the operation can be very difficult, and the prognosis is very poor.

## 2.  Fistula

Gastrointestinal fistulae are seen commonly in the later stages of management of infected pancreatic necrosis. Most fistulas are secondary to focal colonic necrosis and, if necessary, are managed by simple defunctioning ileostomy, which we perform through a small incision. More extensive colonic necrosis presents as catastrophic worsening of MODS, but in our experience, this complication is very rare unless open necrosectomy has been carried out.

Duodenal and gastric fistulae can be managed conservatively, although a period of TPN may be required. Pancreatic fistulae are expected after percutaneous necrosectomy. Patients with pancreatic fistulae may be sent home with a soft catheter in place to be removed in the outpatient clinic when drainage stops, usually within 3–4 weeks. Persistent fistulae may necessitate pancreatic duct stenting or, rarely, distal pancreatectomy in cases of disconnected duct syndrome.

# Conclusion

Management strategies for patients presenting with acute pancreatitis associated with pancreatic and peri-pancreatic necrosis have changed radically in the last 10 years. Previously held dogma and uncompromising operative strategies have matured into a complex and dynamic, multi-modal management strategy. Inadequate drainage of sepsis is being recognized as the key to deteriorating organ failure, and ultimately mortality, rather than the previously held belief that infected necrosis demanded a radical approach. General principles, however, remain to avoid any major procedure in a patient with organ dysfunction and to delay intervention where possible to allow organization of the necrosis, when morbidity and mortality are minimal.

## Selected Readings

Ayub K, Imada R, Slavin J (2004) Endoscopic retrograde cholangiopan-creatography in gallstone-associated acute pancreatitis. Cochrane Database Syst Rev CD003630

Balthazar EJ (2002) Acute pancreatitis: assessment of severity with clinical and CT evaluation. Radiology 223:603–613

Buchler M, Uhl W, Beger HG (1993) Surgical strategies in acute pancreatitis. Hepatogastroenterology 40:563–568

Buter A, Imrie CW, Carter CR, et al. (2002) Dynamic nature of early organ dysfunction determines outcome in acute pancreatitis. Br J Surg 89:298–302

Carter CR, McKay CJ, Imrie CW (2000) Percutaneous necrosectomy and sinus tract endoscopy in the management of infected pancreatic necrosis: an initial experience. Ann Surg 232:175–180

Johnson CD, Abu-Hilal M (2004) Persistent organ failure during the first week as a marker of fatal outcome in acute pancreatitis. Gut 53:1340–1344

Lankisch PG, Lerch MM (2006) The role of antibiotic prophylaxis in the treatment of acute pancreatitis. J Clin Gastroenterol 40:149–155

Marik PE, Zaloga GP (2004) Meta-analysis of parenteral nutrition versus enteral nutrition in patients with acute pancreatitis. BMJ 328:1407

McKay CJ, Imrie CW (2004) The continuing challenge of early mortality in acute pancreatitis. Br J Surg 91:1243–1244

# 2
# Acute Pancreatitis

**José Eduardo M. Cunha, Marcel C.C. Machado, and José Jukemura**

## Pearls and Pitfalls

- Acute pancreatitis (AP) represents a spectrum of disease ranging from a mild, self-limited course to a rapidly progressive, severe illness.
- Most patients have a mild disease and recover without specific treatment, whereas the mortality rate of the severe form, which occurs in about 10–15% of patients, exceeds 20%. Clinical severity is determined by the degree of pancreatic and peripancreatic necrosis defined by contrast-enhanced computed tomography (CT).
- The most common causes are gallstones and alcohol abuse.
- The diagnosis of AP requires two of the following three features: characteristic abdominal pain, hyperamylasemia, and findings of AP on CT.
- Management of mild AP is supportive – intravenous fluids and analgesics; severe pancreatitis requires management in an intensive care unit.
- Early enteral nutrition is the preferred feeding method in severe AP, because it preserves the intestinal mucosal barrier and does not predispose to fungal infections.
- Early endoscopic retrograde cholangiography with sphincterotomy is indicated for severe biliary pancreatitis and cholangitis.

K.I. Bland et al. (eds.), *Surgery of the Pancreas and Spleen*, DOI: 10.1007/978-1-84996-369-5_2, © Springer-Verlag London Limited 2011

- CT or US-guided fine-needle aspiration (FNA) for bacteriology should be performed in patients suspected of having infected pancreatic necrosis.
- Necrosectomy as opposed to catheter drainage is recommended for infected pancreatic necrosis.
- Newer, minimal access methods (percutaneous, laparoscopic, endoscopic, and small incision, focused open necrosectomy) have been introduced recently.
- Early operative intervention within 14 days of onset of AP is discouraged for necrotizing pancreatitis (NP).
- Sterile pancreatic necrosis should be managed conservatively.

## Introduction

Acute pancreatitis (AP) is an acute inflammatory disease of the pancreas with an incidence that varies from 15 to 80 cases per year per 100,000 adults depending on the world region. According to recent data, the USA and Brazil are the countries with the highest occurrence rates. The clinical manifestations and evolution of AP depend on the various etiologic and morphologic aspects. Approximately 80–85% of patients have a mild, self-limiting process associated with edema in the interstitial pancreatic tissue or around the gland; this interstitial edematous pancreatitis resolves with supportive medical management. The remaining 15–20% of patients present with a severe, potentially life-threatening form of the disease; necrotizing pancreatitis is characterized by pancreatic parenchymal and/or peripancreatic necrosis which is generally associated with single or multiple organ failure (MODS). In these patients, the mortality rate approaches 30%.

## Etiology

Many factors play an etiologic role in AP. The most common etiologic factors are outlined in Table 2.1, the most common of which are alcohol abuse and gallstones.

TABLE 2.1. Etiology of acute pancreatitis.

Gallstone disease

Alcohol

Metabolic

    Hyperlipidemia

    Hypercalcemia

Iatrogenic

    Endoscopic retrograde cholangiopancreatography

    Abdominal and non-abdominal operations

Neoplasms

    Periampullary cancer

    Intraductal pancreatic mucinous tumors

*Pancreas divisum*

Genetic

    Cystic fibrosis

    Hereditary pancreatitis

Infectious and parasitic agents

    Viruses (Mumps, Coxsackie B and HIV)

    Bacteria (*Salmonella* and *Shigella* species)

    Biliary parasites (*Ascaris lumbricoides*)

Medications (anti-inflammatory, antimicrobial, diuretics, immunosuppressants)

Trauma

Vasculitis (Systemic lupus erythematosus and polyarteritis nodosa)

Toxins (Scorpion venom)

# Pathophysiology

Intracellular activation of trypsinogen into trypsin within the acinar cell is an important initiating event in most forms of the disease. The subsequent activation of other pancreatic proenzymes such as proelastase, chymotrypsinogen, procarboxypeptidase and pyrophospholipase $A_2$ by auto activation of trypsin leads to pancreatic acinar cell damage with spillage of activated enzymes into the pancreatic and peripancreatic tissues. Previous theories involving intraductal activation of enzymes within the pancreatic duct, reflux of bile, ductal hypertension, and a ductal rupture have been disproven. It appears that all etiologies of necrotizing pancreatitis work via this final common pathway, even alcohol abuse, biliary tract obstruction, and other etiologic factors. The prognosis of the AP depends on the intensity of the multiple organ dysfunction syndrome (MODS) caused by the systemic inflammatory response (SIRS). The pathogenesis of the systemic manifestations of complicated AP seems to result from release of multiple inflammatory mediators from activated leukocytes and macrophages, including the pro-inflammatory cytokines IL-1, IL-6, IL-8, PAF, and TNF-alpha, which apparently play the key roles in initiating the septic syndrome. The anti-inflammatory cytokines IL-10, TNF-soluble receptors, and IL1 receptor antagonist are also implicated in this inflammatory response to AP to some extent.

Infection of the necrotic tissue by enteric microorganisms represents a serious complication of AP that takes place in about 30% of patients with necrotizing pancreatitis.

## Classification of Acute Pancreatitis

A classification system for AP based on clinical, pathologic, and radiologic criteria was proposed at an international symposium held in Atlanta in 1992. This "Atlanta classification" defined severe AP based on clinical manifestations, high scores in multiple factor scoring systems, as well as evidence of organ failure and intrapancreatic pathology. Although the Atlanta classification represented an important step forward in the understanding and management of AP, new knowledge achieved recently on pathophysiology, diagnosis, and management of AP have made some of its aspects outdated.

These factors motivated the organization of an international study group that is involved currently in revising and updating the classification of AP.

## Clinical Presentation

Abdominal pain of moderate to severe intensity is the initial symptom in the majority of the patients. Abdominal pain generally presents as sudden onset and persists for one or more days with nausea and vomiting present in about 90% of patients. Fever is a common finding over the first several days; however, it usually resolves thereafter. When present after the second week in patients with necrotizing pancreatitis, fever is usually due to infection of the necrotic tissue. Jaundice is uncommon, although small increases in serum bilirubin may occur due to distal common bile duct compression by the inflamed pancreatic head or when the AP is secondary to a gallstone impacted at the ampulla of Vater.

Severe AP evolves over three variable phases. The first phase involves the first week or two after onset of AP. Clinical manifestations may include fever, leukocytosis, hemodynamic instability, respiratory failure, renal dysfunction, and sensorial disturbances, related to SIRS; the pancreatic and peripancreatic necrosis is usually sterile during this first phase. The second phase often occurs after resolution of SIRS with a period of relative disease and symptom quiescence lasting one to two weeks. During this second phase, the necrosis becomes "superinfected" in up to 30% of patients with necrotizing AP. The third phase evolves along one of three forms. One form leads to liquefaction necrosis and eventual resolution of symptoms and the necrosis over the next 4–12 weeks. A second form involves the organization of sterile, non-infected pancreatic and peripancreatic liquefaction necrosis that persists, causing a feeling of unwell and inability to eat related to the mass effect of this "organized" necrosis which is termed "walled off pancreatic necrosis"; in some type of operative intervention is usually needed to resolve this form. The third form is the most serious and involves progression of the superinfection of the necrosis into a pancreatic abscess with both local and systemic symptoms. Active operative or, if the process is more localized, percutaneous or minimal access intervention with necrosectomy is necessary.

## Risk Factors for Pancreatic Infection

Pancreatic infection occurs in up to 30% of all patients with severe AP. Infection is more likely to occur in patients with extensive pancreatic necrosis. Nevertheless, patients may still become infected even when lesser amounts of the gland are necrotic; indeed, about 20% of patients with necrotizing pancreatitis have primarily peripancreatic necrosis which can become infected. Another risk factor for infection of the pancreatic necrosis is the duration of the disease: the rate of infected necrosis usually increases from the second to the third week, declining to a lesser infection rate after the fourth week.

## Biochemical Diagnosis

Diagnosis of AP is made on the basis of clinical presentation, characterized by the characteristic abdominal pain of pancreatic origin combined with blood tests and imaging modalities. Determination of amylase and/or lipase in plasma remains the gold standard for the diagnosis of AP. Plasma levels of both enzymes peak within the first 24 h of symptoms. Because amylase and lipase have different half-lives, plasma amylase levels remain increased for approximately 36 h, whereas lipase will be sustained for a much longer period. Plasma levels of these enzymes do not correlate with severity of AP.

## Imaging Diagnosis

*Ultrasonography (US)*: Transabdominal US represents the first imaging technique usually utilized for evaluating patients with AP but plays only a limited role in the diagnosis or staging, because the pancreas may not be visible in many patients with AP due to overlying abdominal gas. US can be of value in demonstrating biliary sludge or stones in the gallbladder, thereby implying an etiology of gallstone pancreatitis. US can detect an increased pancreatic volume, changes of the pancreatic parenchyma, and presence of peripancreatic fluid collections. Because US cannot assess organ perfusion, detection of pancreatic necrosis is difficult. This limitation has been addressed by the recent development of echo-enhancers that have made possible a better evaluation of the pancreatic blood supply.

*Computed tomography (CT)*: Contrast-enhanced CT has three major roles in patients with suspected AP: (1) to confirm the diagnostic suspicion, (2) to evaluate severity of the inflammatory process, and (3) to detect complications of the disease, such as pancreatic abscess and pancreatic necrosis. Diagnostic signs of severe AP on CT include pancreatic swelling (Fig. 2.1a), peripancreatic infiltrates, fluid collections and fat necrosis (Figs. 2.1b and 2.2a), and areas of non-enhancement of the pancreas, indicative of parenchymal necrosis (Fig. 2.2b). Abnormal extraluminal gas bubbles on CT are pathognomonic of pancreatic infection (Fig. 2.3). Overall, the accuracy of contrast-enhanced CT for the diagnosis of pancreatic necrosis is 95%. Because no published data supports routine use of CT within the first 24 h of admission in patients with AP, our policy is to perform CTs in patients with severe disease who do not improve after 3–4 days of conservative therapy, and in those whose condition deteriorates after treatment. CT-directed fine needle aspiration is used to obtain pancreatic specimens for microbiologic examination to detect the presence of bacterial contamination in pancreatic necrosis. Rarely, CT may be needed to make the diagnosis in a patient in whom the diagnosis of an abdominal catastrophe requiring emergent celiotomy cannot be excluded.

*Magnetic resonance imaging (MRI)*: MRI is comparable to CT in providing information about the severity of AP and may be superior to CT in demonstrating necrotic debris

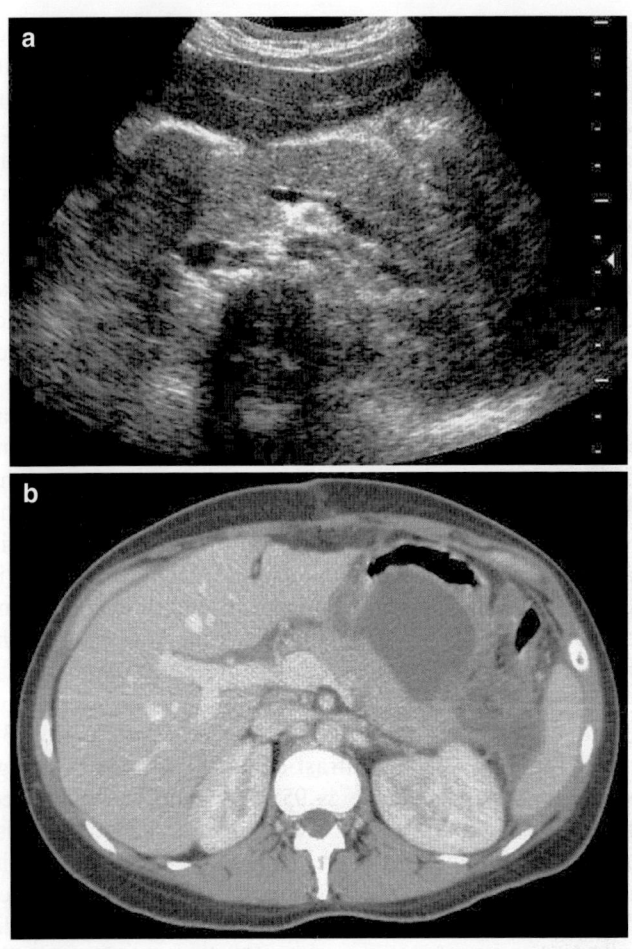

FIGURE 2.1. Mild acute pancreatitis. (a) Ultrasound shows diffuse
enlarged pancreas. (b) Post-contrast CT image shows a lesser sac
acute fluid collection.

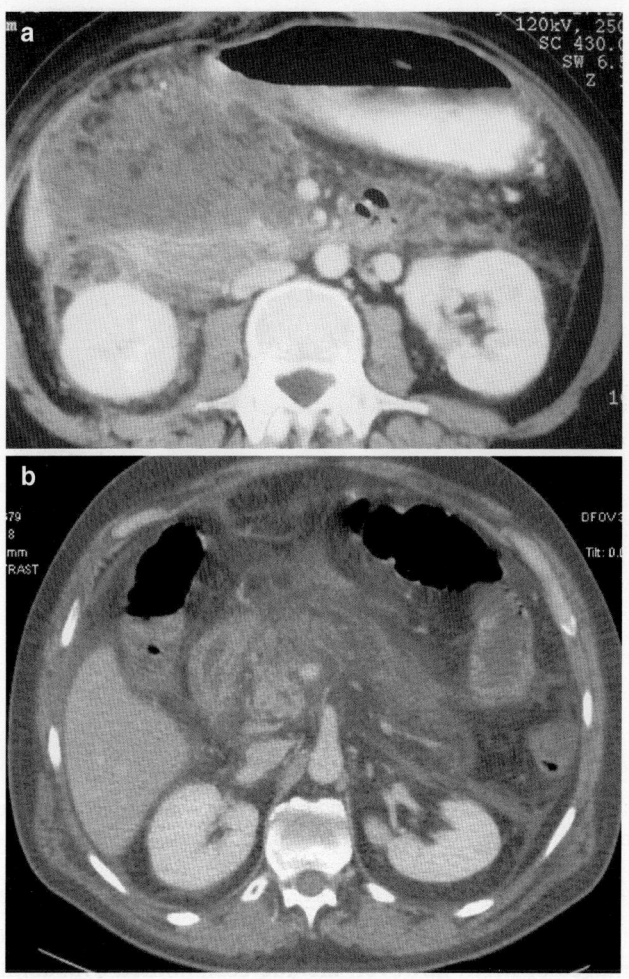

FIGURE 2.2. Severe acute pancreatitis. (**a**) Post-contrast CT shows extensive peripancreatic fat necrosis. (**b**) Partial necrosis of the tail of the pancreas and inflammatory changes in the peripancreatic fat extending to the mesocolon.

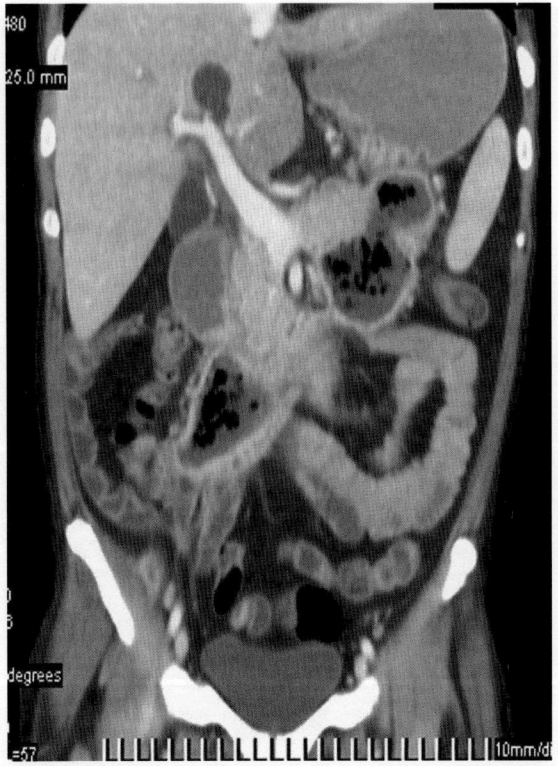

FIGURE 2.3. Coronal volume rendering CT reconstruction. Infected pancreatic necrosis with abnormal gas bubbles.

within peripancreatic fluid collections (Fig. 2.4). The disadvantages of MRI, however, include cost, limited availability, lack of radiologic experience, and the practical difficulties of scanning patients who require ICU monitoring.

*Endoscopic retrograde cholangiopancreatography (ERCP)*: ERCP can be an important tool for diagnosis and therapy in acute and recurrent pancreatitis. Its role in AP is limited to ERC with searching for and treating choledocholithiasis; injection of the pancreatic duct (pancreatography) is usually contraindicated in early days of AP. Less risky techniques,

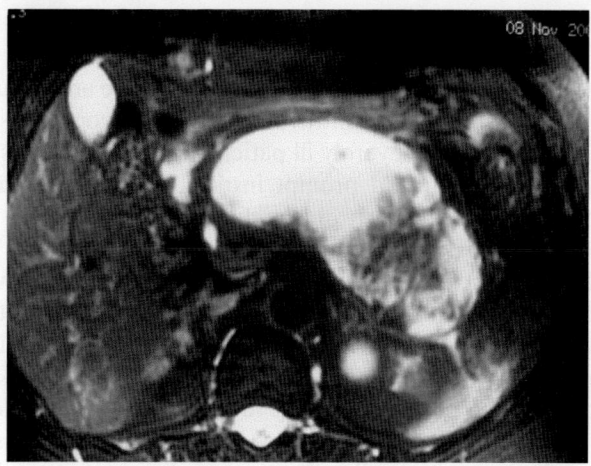

FIGURE 2.4. Axial T2 MR image demonstrates extensive parenchymal necrosis and debris at the body of the pancreas.

including EUS and MRCP, should be considered for diagnosis in these ill patients, saving ERCP for more therapeutic measures, because ERCP can exacerbate the pancreatitis. Routine ERCP is not recommended for patients with mild, acute biliary pancreatitis; cholecystectomy should occur with intraoperative cholangiography.

## Diagnosis of Infection

Recognition of infected pancreatic necrosis can be difficult when based only on clinical grounds. CT usually cannot differentiate "sterile" from "infected" necrosis unless there is extraluminal gas. Fine needle aspiration (FNA) is a reliable, safe procedure to determine bacterial contamination of necrosis. Although in some centers FNA is performed routinely in patients with necrosis and fluid collections, we limit FNA to those patients who exhibit a septic picture and an unfavorable clinical evolution.

## Severity Assessment

Most patients with AP have a self-limiting course and require only general support and intravenous fluids. In contrast, success of treatment of severely ill patients with AP depends on early identification and prompt institution of prophylactic antibiotic treatment. Early objective measures of severity are useful to recognize such patients.

*Multiple factor scoring systems*: The Ranson criteria, developed in 1974, evaluate 11 clinical and laboratory parameters gathered during the first 48 h after the onset of AP. Although this scoring system selects patients who are at a high risk of life-threatening complications, it requires 48 h to complete. The Glasgow criteria, proposed to simplify the Ranson approach, was an equally effective predictor of mortality, regardless of etiology, but its accuracy was no better than the Ranson criteria and also requires 48 h for maximum efficiency. The APACHE II illness grading system has been used more successfully to stage the severity of illness in patients with AP. A score > 6 at admission tends to identify most of patients with severe pancreatitis and has proved useful in many randomized studies to select patients at highest risk. In addition, APACHE II can be employed throughout the course of the disease to follow progression and response to therapy. One disadvantage of APACHE II is that it gives too heavy a weighting for age. Because obesity is a known risk factor for patients with AP, proposal of the APACHE-O score, which scores one extra point for BMI 25–30 and two points for BMI > 30 enhances the accuracy of APACHE II grading of severity.

*CT grading systems*: Because non-enhancing, hypoperfused areas within the pancreas on contrast-enhanced CT correlates with pancreatic necrosis, CT can also be used as a tool for grading of severity in AP. The morphologic severity of AP using the CT Severity Index (CTSI) was developed by Balthazar and coworkers. The CTSI is based on a combination of peripancreatic inflammation, phlegmon, and degree of pancreatic necrosis seen on the initial CT. Large amounts of ischemic or infarcted pancreas obtain the highest scores. In our experience, CT findings of necrosis in the retropancreatic, intercaval-aortic, and the peri-mesenteric vessels are associated with a higher mortality. One limitation is the high cost of repeated CTs related to the need for repeated CTs as the dynamic disease process unfolds.

*Markers of pancreatic injury*: Numerous studies have searched for a blood test that could be performed quickly to discriminate between mild and severe AP. Plasma levels of amylase and lipase have no value in prediction of severity. C-reactive protein (CRP) is the cheapest, most useful (albeit non-pancreas specific) marker to distinguish between edematous and necrotizing AP. Values > 150 mg/l are suggestive of severe AP. Although IL-6, IL-8, and procalcitonin are more sensitive tests than CRP, none of these blood studies are available widely and suspicion of the diagnosis of necrotizing pancreatitis is generally based on clinical and imaging assessment.

## Medical Treatment

Although the majority of patients with AP have an uneventful course, every patient should be treated aggressively until the severity of the disease has been properly determined.

*Supportive care*: The goals of initial management include fluid and electrolyte replacement, nutritional support, and correction of hypovolemia. Some patients should be monitored by measurement of CVP, urine output, and placement of a Swan-Ganz catheter in patients with cardiopulmonary disease or cardiopulmonary decompensation. Good experimental evidence supports the value of aggressive resuscitation and hydration in treatment of AP.

*Analgesic therapy*: The treatment of pain in AP is essential. Moderate and severe pain requires narcotic analgesics, but not morphine, which may cause spasm at the sphincter of Oddi. Patient-controlled analgesia (PCA) via an epidural catheter can be very effective.

*Inhibition of exocrine pancreatic secretion*: Numerous clinical trials have failed to demonstrate any effectiveness of drugs used to inhibit exocrine pancreatic secretion. These data speak against the use of any medication to inhibit pancreatic secretion. Oral intake is withheld by most surgeons during the initial course of the disease.

*Antibiotics*: The value of prophylactic antibiotics in AP remains very controversial. Reduction of infectious complications and mortality has been demonstrated in several but certainly not all randomized studies. Recovery of microorganisms by FNA usually shows polymicrobial, Gram-negative bacteria of intestinal origin and on occasion (~10%) fungal infection, mainly of *Candida* species. Our current policy is to use imipenem and fluconazole in all patients with severe AP.

*Nutritional support*: Patients with severe AP have increased nutritional needs because of increases in energy expenditure and catabolism. Adequate provision of nutrition can be challenging without stimulating pancreatic exocrine secretion. Early enteral feeding is associated with a reduction in the acute phase response and the severity of gut-derived infectious complications of AP.

*Endoscopic treatment*: Currently, most pancreatologists suggest early endoscopic treatment of patients with severe acute biliary pancreatitis. A meta-analysis of four randomized controlled trials of endoscopic sphincterotomy (ES) showed reduced complications and mortality in those patients with biliary obstruction and/or cholangitis [6]. Our policy is to recommend early ES (within 72 h of hospital admission) in patients with severe AP when jaundice and/or cholangitis persists or when patients with initially mild disease deteriorate clinically. ES is of no use in mild biliary AP.

## Surgical Treatment

The role of surgical treatment of AP is to control local complications of the disease.

*Gallstone pancreatitis*: Patients with gallstone pancreatitis not treated previously by ES should be offered same admission cholecystectomy after their pain resolves; recurrent AP occurs in up to 70% of the patients within one year after AP if the gallbladder is not removed. Intraoperative cholangiography should be performed at the time of cholecystectomy. Cholecystectomy should be delayed 3–4 months in patients with severe AP, because early cholecystectomy has a higher complication rate and operative mortality. In patients too ill to undergo cholecystectomy, ES may be an alternative.

*Infected pancreatic necrosis*: Pancreatic infection constitutes the main indication for operative treatment of necrotizing pancreatitis. Failure to recognize and treat these patients results in high mortality rates, whereas the mortality associated with operative debridement and drainage is 10–20%.

Removal of infected pancreatic and peripancreatic necrotic tissue decreases the risks of local and systemic complications. Traditionally, surgical debridement has been performed via an open operative approach via laparotomy. The entire peripancreatic space, including the base of the small bowel mesentery and the paracolic gutters, must be evaluated to effect a complete removal of the necrotic tissue. The CT serves as a guide to all suspect areas of necrosis. Repeat operations may be necessary. When the viability of the transverse colon is compromised, an extended right hemicolectomy with the construction of an ileostomy and mucous fistula is indicated. After completing the necrosectomy, some form of wide peripancreatic drainage should be performed. We have favored partial abdominal closure over multiple Penrose drains and repeat operations every 48–72 h until the completion of necrosis debridement, while others utilize closed irrigation/lavage of the peripancreatic space via inflow and outflow catheters left at the time of necrosectomy.

The results of surgical debridement depend on the timing of the operative procedure. Delaying the initial operation if possible for 3 or 4 weeks after disease onset decreases the mortality, because the necrotic tissue demarcates from viable pancreas, leading to a safer, more complete necrosectomy. Recently, necrosectomy performed by minimally invasive procedures such as laparoscopic and retroperitoneal percutaneous approaches, have been used in selected patients (see chapter 1).

*Sterile pancreatic necrosis (SPN)*: In 60–70% of patients with necrotizing pancreatitis, the necrotic tissue remains sterile. The optimal approach in these patients who are symptomatic is controversial. Some groups suggest that surgical debridement speeds recovery, but many patients can be successfully managed non-operatively. Furthermore, operative intervention may induce bacterial contamination of sterile necrosis with subsequent increase of mortality rates. Nevertheless, progressive deterioration from SIRS and ongoing sepsis are accepted indications for necrosectomy in patients with SPN.

# Selected Readings

Bradley EL III (1991) Operative management of acute pancreatitis: ventral open packing. Hepatogastroenterology 38:134–138

Bradley EL III (1993) A clinically based classification system for acute pancreatitis. Summary of the International Symposium on Acute Pancreatitis, September 11–13, 1992, Atlanta, GA. Arch Surg 128: 586–590

Buchler MW, Gloor B, Muller CA, et al. (2000) Acute necrotizing pancreatitis: treatment strategy according to the status of infection. Ann Surg 232:619–626

Cunha JEM, Machado MCC, Penteado S, et al. (1994) Pan-creatic necrosis in Brazil. In: Bradley EL III (ed) Acute pancreatitis: diagnosis and treatment. Raven, New York, pp 121–125

Garg PK, Khanna S, Bohidar NP, et al. (2001) Incidence, spectrum and antibiotic sensitivity pattern of bacterial infections among patients with acute pancreatitis. J Gastroenterol Hepatol 16:1055–1059

Rau B, Pralle U, Mayer JM, Beger HG (1998) Role of ultra-sonographically guided fine-needle aspiration cytology in the diagnosis of infected pancreatic necrosis. Br J Surg 85:179–184

Sharma VK, Howden CW (1999) Meta-analysis of randomized controlled trials of endoscopic retrograde cholangiography and endoscopic sphincterotomy for the treatment of acute biliary pancreatitis. Am J Gastroenterol 94:3211–3214

Uomo G, Visconti M, Manes G, et al. (1996) Nonsurgical treatment of acute necrotizing pancreatitis. Pancreas 12:142–148

# 3
# Chronic Pancreatitis: From Endotherapy to Surgery

**Jens Werner and Markus W. Büchler**

## Pearls and Pitfalls

- The etiology of chronic pancreatitis is multifactorial with about 65–70% of the cases being attributed to alcohol abuse.
- Multiple hypotheses exist to explain the pathophysiology in various subgroups of patients with chronic pancreatitis, but to date there is no single unifying theory.
- Clinically, there are three stages of the disease: (1) *Stage A* - early stage, recurrent acute attacks with only mild impairment of pancreatic function, (2) *Stage B* - occurrence of disease complications, increasing pain and impaired pancreatic function, (3) *Stage C* - advanced end stage disease, less intense pain with exocrine and endocrine pancreatic insufficiency.
- The diagnosis of chronic pancreatitis is based on a combination of history and physical examination, laboratory data, and imaging, including CT, MRI, ERP, and EUS.
- The management of chronic pancreatitis includes conservative, endoscopic, and surgical approaches.
- Conservative medical treatment is the first line therapy in patients with painful chronic pancreatitis; pancreatic enzyme supplements can abolish protein malabsorption, but steatorrhea cannot be reversed completely; relief of pain is unpredictable.

K.I. Bland et al. (eds.), *Surgery of the Pancreas and Spleen*, DOI: 10.1007/978-1-84996-369-5_3,
© Springer-Verlag London Limited 2011

- A subgroup of patients can profit from endoscopic stenting with permanent regression of the stenosis after stent removal. Endoscopic therapy should be performed as first line therapy in patients with acute cholestasis before carrying out biliodigestive surgery.
- Endoscopic treatment of pseudocysts can be attempted in all symptomatic cysts apart from those with intra-cystic hemorrhage.
- In contrast, long-term pain relief and increase of body weight are better in patients with painful, obstructive chronic pancreatitis when treated operatively.
- Pancreatic head resections, either as a duodenum-preserving pancreatic head resection (DPPHR) or a pancreatoduodenectomy, are usually superior to simple drainage operations. The different variations of DPPHR decrease postoperative morbidity and mortality, maintain exocrine and endocrine function better, and confer a superior quality of life.

## Etiology and Pathophysiology

Chronic pancreatitis is a progressive, destructive inflammatory process that ends in destruction of the pancreatic parenchyma resulting in malabsorption, diabetes mellitus, and severe pain. The etiology of chronic pancreatitis is probably multifactorial. About 65–70% of patients have a history of alcohol abuse, the remaining patients are classified as idiopathic chronic pancreatitis (20–25%), including tropical pancreatitis, a major cause of childhood chronic pancreatitis in tropical regions, or unusual causes including hereditary pancreatitis, cystic fibrosis, and chronic pancreatitis-associated metabolic and congenital factors (Table 3.1). Current evidence suggests that a combination of predisposing factors, including environmental, toxic, and genetic, are involved in most patients rather than one single factor. The best known hypotheses about the pathogenesis of chronic pancreatitis include necrosis-fibrosis,

TABLE 3.1.  Chronic pancreatitis: etiology and pathogenesis.

| Etiology/mechanism of injury | Pathogenesis |
| --- | --- |
| **Toxic metabolic** | |
| Alcohol-induced (genetic mutations) | Toxic-metabolic hypothesis |
| Tobacco | Necrosis-fibrosis |
| Hypercalcemia (hyperparathyroidism) | Protein plug obstructive hypothesis |
| Lipoprotein lipase deficiency | Oxidative stress |
| Apolipoprotein C-2 deficiency | (Detoxification insufficiency) |
| Protein deficiency | |
| Trace element deficiency | |
| Dietary toxins | |
| Medication (phenacetin) | |
| **Idiopathic causes** | Necrosis-fibrosis |
| Early onset | Protein-plug |
| Late onset | |
| Tropical forms | |
| **Genetic** | Necrosis-fibrosis |
| Hereditary | |
|   Autosomal dominant mutations Cationic trypsinogen gene (PRSS1) | |
|   Autosomal-recessive mutations SPINK1, Cationic.trypsinogen | |
| Cystic fibrosis transmembrane conductant regulator (CFTR) defects | |
| α1-antitripsin deficiency | |
| **Autoimmune/Immunologic causes** | Large duct |
| Viral infection (Hepatitis B, Coxsackie) | |

(*continued*)

TABLE 3.1.  (continued).

| Etiology/mechanism of injury | Pathogenesis |
| --- | --- |
| Autoimmune diseases | |
|    Primary autoimmune pancreatitis (AIP) | |
|    Associated with Sjögren's syndrome, Crohn's disease, etc. | |
| **Recurrent and severe AP** | Necrosis-fibrosis |
| Vascular disease | |
| Ischemia | |
| Post-radiation therapy | |
| **Obstructive mechanical causes** | Stone and duct obstruction |
| Pancreas divisum with dysfunctional accessory papilla | Protein-plug |
| Annular pancreas | |
| Papillary stenosis | |
| Pancreatic ductal scarring | |
| Duodenal obstruction (diverticulum, afferent limb syndrome) | |
| Ductal stricture after severe pancreatitis or trauma | |
| Pancreatic ductal stones | |
| Choledochocele | |

toxic-metabolic, oxidative stress, plug and stone formation with duct obstruction, and primary duct obstruction. Repeated episodes of inflammation initiated by autodigestion, one or more episodes of severe pancreatitis, oxidative stress, and/or toxic-metabolic factors lead to activation and continued stimulation of parenchymal pancreatic stellate cells. These stellate cells cause the fibrosis characteristic of chronic pancreatitis. Nevertheless, multiple hypotheses exist to explain the pathophysiology in the various subgroups of patients with chronic pancreatitis, but to date there is no single unifying theory.

# Clinical Presentation

Although abdominal pain is the most common presenting symptom of chronic pancreatitis, pain may be absent in up to 15% of patients with alcohol-related chronic pancreatitis and in up to 20% of patients with non-alcoholic chronic pancreatitis. Steatorrhea is a later symptom, because 90% of exocrine function must be lost before steatorrhea develops. Patients can, however, have symptoms of bloating discomfort (from the steatorrhea), abdominal pain, or change in bowel habits when 60–90% of the pancreatic function is lost. Chronic pancreatitis is a dynamic disease characterized by progressive loss of pancreatic parenchyma caused by inflammation, tissue destruction, and fibrosis. According to Amman, the course of the disease can be classified into three different stages (Table 3.2): *Stage A*: early stage, characterized by recurrent acute attacks, with only mild or no impairment of pancreatic function; *Stage B*: later in the course of the disease, complications occur (pseudocysts, cholestasis, segmental portal hypertension), increasing pain (more frequent acute attacks, increasing pain intensity), impaired pancreatic function; and *Stage C*: end stage disease, characterized by less frequent episodes and less intense pain ("burn out of the pancreas"), with marked impairment of pancreatic function (exocrine and/or endocrine). In all stages of the disease, clinical symptoms (pain, weight loss, steatorrhea, diabetes mellitus, local complications) can be observed in various combinations and degrees.

# Diagnosis

The diagnosis of chronic pancreatitis is based on a thorough history and physical examination, laboratory data, and imaging studies which reflect the imaging abnormalities as well as functional impairments of the pancreas. Chronic pancreatitis is a well-defined disease on histopathologic grounds, but histology is rarely available for diagnosis. The correct diagnosis of chronic pancreatitis is easy in the late stages but difficult in

TABLE 3.2. Chronic pancreatitis: Clinical and morphologic presentation, diagnostic procedures.

| Stage | Clinical picture | | Morphology | Pancreatic function | Diagnostic procedures |
|---|---|---|---|---|---|
| | Pain | Complications | | | |
| **A** Early | Recurrent acute attacks | No complications | Morphologic changes detectable with imaging procedures | Normal pancreatic endocrine and exocrine function | EUS, ERP, MRP, CT |
| **B** Moderate | Increasing pain (number of attacks, intensity, frequency) | Pseudocysts, cholestasis, segmental portal hypertension | Progressive morphologic changes, detectable in several imaging procedures | Impairment of pancreatic function, but rarely steatorrhea | Transabdominal ultrasonography, ERP/MRP, EUS, CT, fasting blood glucose, oral glucose tolerance test |
| **C** Advanced | Decreasing pain ("burn out of the pancreas") | Pseudocysts, cholestasis, segmental portal hypertension | Ductal calculi and parenchymal calcification | Marked impairment of pancreatic function, steatorrhea; diabetes mellitus | Transabdominal ultrasonography, ERP/MRP, CT, fecal elastase, pancreolaurin test, fasting blood glucose, (oral glucose tolerance test) |

early stages of the disease. There are several imaging methods for patients with known or suspected chronic pancreatitis (Table 3.2). In early stages of the disease, both endoscopic retrograde pancreatography (ERP) and endoscopic ultrasonography (EUS) are methods with reliable diagnostic accuracy. Initial studies have shown superiority of EUS (in experienced centers) over ERP for the diagnosis of chronic pancreatitis in its early stages. Transabdominal ultrasonography (US) is less sensitive for the diagnosis of chronic pancreatitis and should be limited generally to patients with advanced stages. In patients with early stages, we believe that the combination of ERP and CT provide the most reliable morphologic information. An alternative diagnostic method is EUS. Among all imaging methods, MRI (magnetic resonance imaging) and MRCP (magnetic resonance cholangiopancreatography) is the method with the most rapid development over the last years. With further improvement of hardware and software, it is likely that these methods will be able to visualize even the early stages of the disease in the near future. The most common pancreatic function tests do not detect mild to moderate exocrine pancreatic insufficiency with adequate accuracy. Therefore, pancreatic function tests play only a complementary role in the routine clinical evaluation of chronic pancreatitis; however, these tests are important methods used in clinical research or specialized pancreatic disease centers.

## Treatment

The treatment of chronic pancreatitis is complex and should involve conservative, endoscopic, and operative therapeutic approaches. The primary treatment of chronic pancreatitis is addressed not at the disease itself but rather at the complications of the disease: abdominal pain, maldigestion, diabetes, pseudocyst, splenic vein thrombosis with gastric varicies and bleeding, bile duct obstruction, duodenal obstruction, and pancreatic cancer. Appropriate management requires individualization in almost every patient. A complication of chronic pancreatitis managed medically in one patient may be best handled by operative intervention in another patient because of confounding factors. Thus, treatment of chronic pancreatitis requires a cooperative, multidisciplinary team.

## Conservative Treatment

The main goals of treatment of chronic pancreatitis involve management of steatorrhea, malnutrition, and pain. About 80% of the patients with chronic pancreatitis can be managed by dietary alterations and pancreatic enzyme supplements; 10–15% of patients need oral supplements (polymeric or semi-elemental), 5% need enteral tube feeding, and around 1% will need total parenteral nutrition. Decrease in steatorrhea and supplementation of absorbable calories are the main goal of nutritional therapy in chronic pancreatitis. Treatment of exocrine insufficiency starts with dietary recommendations and pancreatic enzyme supplementation. Total abstinence from alcohol and frequent meals are the basics for dietary recommendations. When weight loss and/or steatorrhea(15 g/d) develop, oral supplementation with effective pancreatic enzyme preparations is indicated. Furthermore, malabsorption of proteins and carbohydrates, meteorism (gaseous distention), and diarrhea are also clinical indications. The main goal of the treatment of pancreatic exocrine dysfunction is to ensure that optimal amounts of lipase reach the duodenum together with the delivered food. With the currently available pancreatic enzyme preparations, azotorrhea (protein malabsorption) can be abolished, while steatorrhea can usually be reduced but not totally corrected.

Pain is a major problem. While pain may also be treated by invasive interventional or operative techniques, medical treatment is generally the first line therapy in patients with painful chronic pancreatitis. The pathogenic mechanisms of pain influence the therapeutic approach. Two mechanisms have been suggested for the generation of pain in the absence of local complications – inflammatory changes of pancreatic parenchyma with involvement of intrapancreatic nerves and ductal/parenchymal hypertension. The former has been approached through various analgesics and anti-inflammatory agents but with little success. All attempts at avoiding use of addictive opiates should be the goal; use of narcotic analgesics introduces a new problem of potential chemical dependency which markedly complicates any further treatment. In contrast, approaches to treat the ductal/parenchymal hypertension are invasive (see below).

Besides complete alcohol abstinence to try to prevent further exacerbations of inflammation, there are no specific dietary measures effective in preventing pancreatic pain. Even total abstinence from alcohol achieves pain relief only in about 50% of the patients with moderate to mild chronic pancreatitis. Guidelines for analgesic treatment in patients with chronic pancreatitis are based on the recommendations of the World Health Organization (WHO). One physician should be responsible for the administration of analgesics. For the first step in pain management, non-narcotic agents like acetaminophen or non-steroidal anti-inflammatory drugs (NSAIDs) are recommended. Only when necessary should opiates be used, and all attempts to discontinue opiate usage should be exhausted. Every patient requires individual types and doses of analgesic drugs, starting with the lowest doses necessary to control pain. In patients with pain caused mainly by inflammation and by invasion of inflammatory cells, anti-inflammatory drugs like NSAIDs may be helpful for their both analgesic and anti-inflammatory properties.

## Endoscopic Treatment

Between 40% and 70% of patients with pancreatic pain can be managed effectively by medical treatment. This percentage may increase by the combination of medical therapy and interventional procedures. In patients with pancreatic ductal stenosis and obstructing pancreatic ductal calculi, pancreatic pain can be improved through a combination of endoscopic sphincterotomy, ductal stenting, and lithotripsy. Some studies show a clinically important improvement of pain in patients with successful lithotripsy by experienced interventional endoscopists; other studies have been unable to demonstrate a prolonged benefit. The working theory is that by effectively draining the pancreatic duct into the duodenum, pancreatic ductal hypertension and the associated parenchymal hypertension can be decreased, leading to a decrease in inflammation of the intrapancreatic nerves and improvement in pancreatic pain in some patients; unfortunately, this beneficial effect is often temporary.

*Pseudocysts.* Besides causing pain, pancreatic pseudocysts are associated with other complications, albeit rare ~10%, such as infection, compression of adjacent structures, venous complications, hemorrhage, or rupture into other anatomic cavities (pleural or peritoneal). Endoscopic treatment of pseudocysts probably should be attempted in most all symptomatic cysts with the exception of hemorrhage into a pseudocyst which is a contra-indication.

In contrast to acute pancreatitis, pancreatic pseudocysts are a late complication of chronic pancreatitis. There are three main techniques for endoscopic decompression of pancreatic pseudocysts: transgastric, transduodenal, and transpapillary. The transgastric and the transduodenal approach require a clear bulging of the cyst into the gastric or the duodenal lumen in order to ensure a short distance (<1 cm) between the cystic wall and the intestinal tract. In this context, the role of EUS has been shown to be effective in selected patients in locating the cyst and decreasing the risk of hemorrhage into the cyst.

In the literature, the technical success rate appears better for cystoduodenostomy than for cystogastrostomy, in large part due to a higher complication rate in the latter. Overall, the mortality appears to be almost zero, yet the morbidity ranges between 3% and 11%. A more recent approach is to access (and drain) the cystic cavity indirectly through the papilla and the ductal system. For this treatment, a selective, endoscopic, pancreatic sphincterotomy and a retrograde pancreaticography is necessary to introduce a guidewire into the pancreatic duct and then into the pseudocyst; thereafter, a double pig-tail endoprosthesis can be inserted over the guidewire, through the papilla, and into the cyst. Again, the mortality is low, and the morbidity has been reported to be 2–7%; this approach may be preferable in some patients but requires a very experienced endoscopist. This approach may not always be feasible because of strictures or stones between the papilla and location of the cyst. In this latter case or if there are other contra-indications, the patient should be referred to a surgeon.

*Common bile duct stenosis* is a potential mechanical complication of chronic pancreatitis. The treatment of common bile duct stenosis in patients with chronic pancreatitis often requires a "team approach" between endoscopist and surgeon. The decision for operative intervention depends on the patient's age, comorbidities, course of the chronic pancreatitis, and the etiology of the stricture. There is a subgroup of patients who profit from placement of a non-permanent, plastic stent with eventual resolution of the stenosis after stent removal. A stent should be considered strongly as first line therapy in patients with acute cholestasis before carrying out (biliodigestive) surgery. Similarly for patients who refuse operative treatment or who have significant comorbidities, an endoscopic approach is the initial therapy of choice with good short-and medium-term results. In a prospective follow-up study, Kahl et al. reported that endoscopic drainage of biliary obstruction provides excellent short-term results but only moderate long-term success. Patients without calcifications of the pancreatic head appear to benefit the most from biliary stenting, because the inflammation causing the extrinsic compression may be reversible. In contrast, patients with pancreatic calcifications have an increased risk of failure of a 12 month course of endoscopic stenting because of the associated fibrosis. Major limitations of long-term endobiliary stenting include stent clogging, stent migration, and cholangitis, which occur frequently. Alternatively, self-expandable wall stents may improve the results, but these metal stents which cannot migrate are not able to be removed, and most pancreatologists do not use these stents for benign disease.

Currently, there are no long-term follow-up data to clarify the role of endoscopic approaches (also which stents are preferable) for the management of cholestasis in chronic pancreatitis. Especially in young patients with chronic pancreatitis without any comorbidities precluding operative intervention, definitive therapy for recurrent or persistent cholestasis is best provided by a biliodigestive bypass procedure combined with either a pancreatic ductal drainage procedure or pancreatic resection.

## Operative Treatment

There are several different concepts for the operative treatment of chronic pancreatitis. The concept of preservation of functioning pancreatic parenchyma (*drainage operations*) would be the goal for protection against further loss of pancreatic function. The second main concept is based on *resective procedures* either in the situation where there is no dilation of the pancreatic duct, if the pancreatic head is enlarged, or if a pancreatic carcinoma is suspected in the setting of chronic pancreatitis. These two concepts involve different operative procedures.

*Drainage procedures.* Sphincterotomy of the pancreatic duct was one of the first operative procedures proposed for patients with a dilated pancreatic duct in chronic pancreatitis with presumed obstruction or stenosis at the papilla Vater. Unfortunately, this procedure was associated with minimal lasting success for the amelioration of pain, indicating that a stenosis at the papilla of Vater is not the cause of pain in chronic pancreatitis nor the cause of ductal dilation.

In contrast, direct ductal-enteric drainage by the original Puestow procedure or its modification by Partington and Rochelle is more successful in patients with chronic pancreatitis and a dilated pancreatic duct. The original Puestow procedure included resection of the tail of the pancreas with filleting open the pancreatic duct proximally along the body of the pancreas with anastomosis to a Roux-en-Yloop of jejunum. Partington and Rochelle modified the Puestow procedure by eliminating the resection of the pancreatic tail. A recent procedure in volve sawedge shaped opening of the pancreaticduct (even when the duct is <5 mm) with a subsequent pancreatico-jejunostomy. The preservation of functional tissue and reduction of operative mortality to less than 1% and morbidity to less than 10% are the goals and benefits of this operation. Unfortunately, large series have reported persistence or recurrence of pain at long-term followup (>5 year) in 30–50% of patients; in addition, patients with a dominant mass in the head of the pancreas and a non-dilated pancreatic duct do not appear to profit from a drainage procedure at all. A recent randomized controlled trial demonstrated that operative drainage in selected patients with a large duct was more effective than endoscopic treatment in patients with obstruction of the pancreatic duct.

# Pancreatic Resections

*Pancreatoduodenectomy (Kausch-Whipple procedure).* For many surgeons, a pancreatoduodenectomy is the gold standard for patients with the pain of chronic pancreatitis, although the newer, duodenum-preserving procedures are good (and possibly better) alternatives as well (see below). The approach of resection of the proximal gland is based on Longmire's tenet that the "pacemaker" of pain is in the head of the pancreas. The indications for pancreatoduodenectomy in patients with chronic pancreatitis and pain are: (1) a non-dilated pancreatic duct (diameter <6 mm measured in the body of the gland), (2) an enlarged head of the pancreas, often containing cysts and calcifications, (3) a previous, ineffective ductal drainage procedure, and/or (4) when there is the possibility of malignancy in the head of the gland. This latter subgroup comprises up to 6–10% of patients undergoing operative intervention for chronic pancreatitis.

After pancreatoduodenectomy, >80% of patients have permanent pain relief, which is considerably greater than after a drainage operation. In experienced centers, a pancreatoduodenectomy can be performed with a low operative mortality rate (<2%), and a morbidity of ~40%. Although the classic pancreatoduodenectomy has these advantages, there is some long-term morbidity in chronic pancreatitis patients, especially with regard to quality of life. In addition to development of diabetes, patients experience postoperative digestive dysfunction, including dumping, diarrhea, peptic ulcer, and dyspeptic complaints.

To address these effects of the classic pancreatoduodenectomy which involved a distal gastrectomy, "organ-preserving" operations like the pylorus-preserving pancreatoduodenectomy were introduced (Fig. 3.1). Symptoms of dumping and

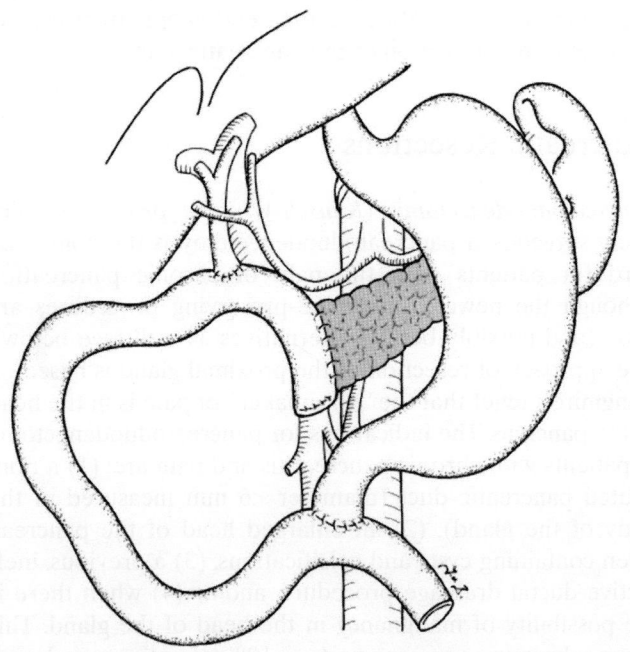

FIGURE 3.1. Pylorus-preserving pancreatoduodenectomy.

bile-reflux gastritis can be decreased by preserving the stomach, the pylorus, and the first part of the duodenum. In addition, regarding quality of life, a pylorus-preserving technique provides better results than the classic pancreatoduodenectomy procedure; weight gain occurs in 90% of the patients postoperatively while still leading to long-lasting pain relief in 85–90% of the patients. Pylorus-preserving resections, however, appear to have a somewhat greater incidence of transient delayed gastric emptying postoperatively (20–30% of the patients) as well as the risk of cholangitis and the long-term occurrence of exocrine and endocrine pancreatic insufficiency (seen in >45% of patients), representing the possible drawbacks of this operation in chronic pancreatitis patients. The relevant studies (level I and II) comparing classic with pylorus-preserving pancreatoduodenectomy could not demonstrate a clear advantage for either resection. One should remember, however, that pancreatoduodenectomy was originally introduced to treat malignant pancreatic or periampullary disease by an oncologic resection. Therefore, for a benign disorder such as chronic pancreatitis, there is no reason – other than the occasional inability to exclude pancreatic cancer definitely – to remove peripancreatic organs (the distal stomach, the duodenum, and the extrahepatic bile ducts), which are involved only secondarily in chronic pancreatitis. This concept stimulated the development of organ-preserving pancreatic resections.

*Duodenum-preserving pancreatic head resection (DPPHR).* This procedure addresses patients with a dominant mass in the head of the pancreas with or without a dilated main pancreatic duct. The duodenum-preserving resection (Beger procedure) includes a ventral dissection and dorsal mobilization of the head of the pancreas. After division of the pancreas anterior to the porto-mesenteric vein (as with a pancreatoduodenectomy), the resection is carried out toward the papilla of Vater. A subtotal resection of the pancreatic head is carried out leaving a small margin of pancreatic tissue associated with the duodenum containing the common bile duct; a small rim of pancreatic tissue toward the vena cava should be preserved as well during removal of most all of the uncinate process. In most patients, it is possible to free the bile duct from the surrounding scarring without disrupting continuity with the ampulla of Vater, thereby avoiding the need for a bilio-digestive anastomosis. In some patients (~20%), the common bile duct is obstructed and should be opened, so that the bile will drain into the cavity of the resected pancreatic head which is drained into a Roux-en-Y limb of jejunum. The standard reconstruction consists of a Roux-en-pancreaticojejunostomy to the distal pancreatic remnant (body and tail of pancreas) and a pancreatojejunostomy to the rim of pancreas at the duodenum (including the opened bile duct if needed). In up to 10% of patients, this DPPHR procedure is combined with a lateral pancreaticoje-junostomy to drain multiple stenoses of the main pancreatic duct. The mortality rate is low (1%), and the morbidity rate is around 15%, less than after pancreatoduodenectomy.

When compared with pancreatoduodenectomy in patients with chronic pancreatitis, the DPPHR offers the advantage of preserving the duodenum and extrahepatic biliary tree, and its superiority over even the pylorus-preserving resection has been shown in prospective studies. Patients who underwent the DPPHR had greater weight gain, a better glucose toler-ance, and a higher capacity for insulin secretion. In long-term follow-up, about 20% of the patients developed new onset of diabetes mellitus, similar to the incidence of diabetes after pancreatoduodenectomy. There is some evidence that endo-crine function may be better preserved after DPPHR when compared with patients with chronic pancreatitis not under-going operation, possibly secondary to the relief of pancreatic ductal obstruction/hypertension.

With regard to pain status, 90% of patients after DPPHR have long-term relief of pain. With regard to quality of life, 69% of the patients in one study were rehabilitated profes-sionally, 26% retired, and only 5% of the patients were unim-proved. Considering the better pain status, a lesser frequency of acute episodes of chronic pancreatitis, especially in those patients with an enlarged pancreatic head, marked decrease in the need for further hospitalization, low early and late mortality rate, and the restoration of a better quality of life, evidence suggests that DPPHR may delay somewhat the natural course of the disease of chronic pancreatitis.

The DPPHR was modified by Frey and colleagues to include a longitudinal pancreatico-jejunostomy combined with a local "coring out" of the pancreatic head without the need for an extensive dissection near the superior mesenteric vessels as with the DPPHR. The Frey and DPPHR have undergone evaluation in multiple comparative trials, confirming their effectiveness as operative procedures for chronic pancreatitis. A modified technique (Bern procedure) of the Beger and Frey procedures has been described recently in patients with chronic pancreatitis (Fig. 3.2). This extended Frey procedure combines the advantages of the Beger and Frey procedure by maintaining a non-anatomic, subtotal central pancreatic head resection but without the need for trans-section of the gland over the superior mesenteric vein (SMV), the most tedious part of the DPPHR procedure which was the major advantage offered by the Frey procedure. This modified technique reduces the risk of intraoperative bleeding which is especially increased in the presence of portal hypertension.

*Left-sided pancreatic resection (distal pancreatectomy)*: Most surgeons believe that the pancreatic head is the pacemaker in chronic pancreatitis, and therefore, pancreatic head resections should be the target for most patients with chronic pancreatitis affecting the entire gland. There is, however, a small and carefully selected group of patients in whom a left-sided pancreatic resection is the appropriate treatment. This subgroup is selected by imaging techniques, including CT, ERCP, or MRI outlining inflammatory complications, such as pseudocysts, fistula, and pancreatic duct stenosis, involving only (or primarily) the body and/or tail region of the pancreas. A good example is the patient who develops a mid-ductal stricture after an episode of necrotizing pancreatitis secondary to gallstone pancreatitis. Similarly, suspicion of a neoplasm or recurrent acute pancreatitis believed secondary to an isolated, mid-ductal

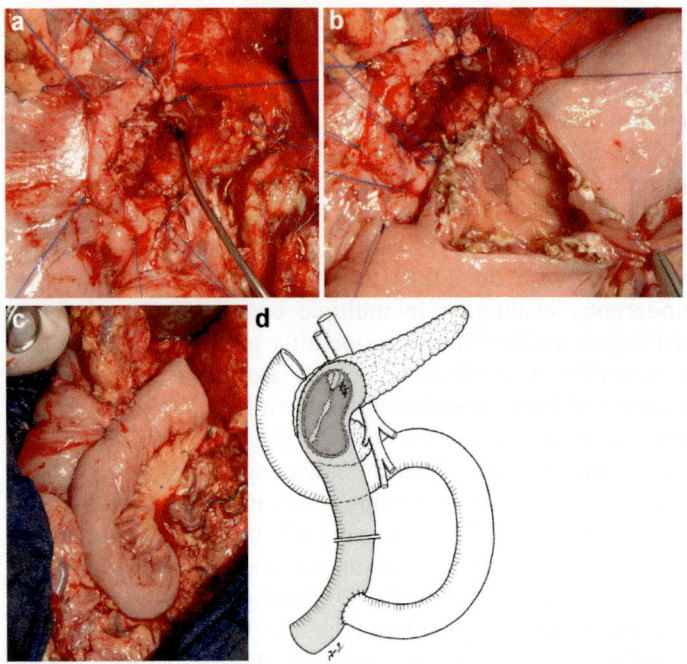

FIGURE 3.2. Bern modification of the duodenum-preserving pancreatic head resection. (**a**) The pancreatic head was resected, and the pancreatic rim sutured with PDS 4-0. The pancreatic duct is cannulated completely to the left. (**b**) Side-to-side pancreaticojejunostomy: The posterior wall is sutured as a double-layer with continuous running sutures. (**c**) The anterior wall of the side-to-side anastomosis is completed. The jejunal loop is brought to the upper abdomen transmesocolically. (**d**) Bern modification of the duodenum preserving pancreatic head resection after reconstruction has been completed.

stricture maybe justification for a left-sided pancreatic resection. Overall, about 10% of all patients who undergo operative intervention for chronic pancreatitis may be candidates for a distal pancreatectomy. These distal pancreatectomies for benign disease can be performed without splenectomy, but conservation of the splenic artery and vein can be difficult and is time-consuming. Nevertheless, the advantage of avoiding the possibility of overwhelming post-splenectomy sepsis should be taken into consideration as well as the importance of the spleen for maintenance of the host defense system. Thus, preservation of the spleen is desirable if there is no clear indication for splenectomy, such as perisplenic pseudocyst or inflammatory/fibrotic encasement of the splenic vessels.

*Central pancreatectomy (middle segmentectomy).* Benign lesions of the neck and proximal body of the pancreas, such as the exceedingly rare *focal chronic pancreatitis* or *post-traumatic pancreatitis*, pose an interesting operative challenge. If the lesions are not amenable to simple enucleation, surgeons may be faced with the choice of performing a right-sided resection (pancreatoduodenectomy) or a left-sided resection (distal pancreatectomy) to include the lesion, resulting in resection of a substantial amount of otherwise functioning pancreatic parenchyma. Central pancreatic resections have been reported primarily for benign or low-grade neoplasms with Roux-en-Y pancreatojejunostomy reconstruction. Central pancreatectomy affords the possibility of saving functional pancreatic tissue in attempt to avoid the complications of pancreatic insufficiency. Further studies, however, must prove the effectiveness of such an operation for patients with chronic pancreatitis. Central resections in patients with chronic pancreatitis must be viewed with caution and considered only in highly selected cases.

Pancreatic resection with islet cell autotransplantation. Because of the concerns of pancreatic endocrine insufficiency after any pancreatic resection for chronic pancreatitis, renewed interest has focused on the possibility of performing a total pancreatectomy, isolating the islets, and reinfusing (*auto*transplanting) the islets into the liver. Improvements in islet cell harvesting and preservation for islet cell *allo*transplantation for diabetics have allowed new enthusiasm in this technique for patients with chronic pancreatitis. Results to date are encouraging, but the inability to harvest reliably an adequate number of islets and to prove successful engraftment within the liver remain current limitations. This approach maybe more effective early in the disease when islets have not been depleted.

## Outcome

The comparison of endoscopic and operative treatment of patients with painful, obstructive chronic pancreatitis demonstrates that long-term pain relief and increase in body weight are better in the operatively treated patients.

Only a few randomized-controlled trials have compared the different operative approaches (Table 3.3). Klempa

TABLE 3.3. Chronic pancreatitis: Randomized-controlled trials comparing different operative techniques of pancreatic resection.

| Author | Operation | n | Results |
|---|---|---|---|
| Klempa et al. 1995 | PD | 21 | DPPHR > PD: pain relief; new onset of diabetes, better weight gain |
| | DPPHR | 22 | DPPHR = PD: mortality and morbidity |
| Büchler et al. 1995 | ppPD | 20 | DPPHR > ppPD: pain, weight gain, endocrine function; |
| | DPPHR | 20 | Morbidity: DPPHR 15% vs. ppPD 20% |
| Müller et al. 1997 | ppPD | 10 | DPPHR > ppPD: delayed gastric emptying |
| | DPPHR | 10 | |
| Makowiec et al. 2004 | ppPD | 44 | DPPHR = ppPD: endocrine function, QoL |
| | DPPHR | 43 | |
| Izbicki et al. 1998 | ppPD | 31 | Frey > ppPD: postoperative complications, QoL |
| | Frey | 30 | Frey = ppPD: pain relief |
| Izbicki et al. 1997 | Frey | 38 | DPPHR = Frey: pain, morbidity, endocrine and exocrine function |
| | DPPHR | 37 | |

PD: classic pancreatoduodenectomy; DPPHR: duodenum-preserving pancreatic head resection; ppPD: pylorus-preserving pancreatoduodenectomy.

and coworkers demonstrated the superiority of duodenum-preserving pancreatic head resection (DPPHR) versus a classic pancreatoduodenectomy with regard to pain relief (100% vs. 70%), as well as a lesser incidence of exocrine insufficiency, better weight gain, and a lesser rate of new onset diabetes (9% vs. 29%). In addition, three randomized trials compared the DPPHR versus a pylorus-preserving pancreatoduodenectomy in chronic pancreatitis (evidence-based Level I data). In the first study, the operation-related morbidity was 15% after DPPHR and 20% after pylorus-preserving resection. Patients who underwent DPPHR had less pain, greater weight gain, better glucose tolerance, and higher insulin secretion capacity 6 months postoperatively. A second trial demonstrated that DPPHR is not associated with delayed gastric emptying postoperatively as was the pylorus-preserving pancreatoduodenectomy. In contrast, the third trial, while showing comparability of the two operations, was unable to demonstrate any difference between the two techniques with regard to exocrine and endocrine function.

Two other evidence-based, Level I studies compared the Beger procedure and pylorus-preserving pancreatoduodenectomy with the Frey procedure. The Frey procedure had less postoperative complications (19% vs. 53%), an overall better quality of life, and an equivalent relief of pain compared with a pylorus-preserving pancreatoduodenectomy. On the other hand, the two variations of the DPPHR, the Beger and Frey procedures, were similar with regard to morbidity, pain relief, and preservation of exocrine and endocrine function. Thus, in many centers, one form of DHPPR (either the Beger or Frey procedure) has become the technique of choice for pancreatic head resection in chronic pancreatitis.

In summary, definite evidence for the best operative method for treating painful chronic pancreatitis is still not fully accepted. The study designs in the few randomized controlled trials (evidence-based Level I data) available today have some limitations in design and reporting of morbidity and include only small numbers of patients. Nevertheless, the different variations of the DPPHR, Beger, Frey, and Bern procedures appear to be as equally successful in achieving long-term pain control as pancreatoduodenectomy, but they have fewer postoperative complications and appear to be superior with regard to preservation of pancreatic function and quality of life.

# Selected Readings

Ammann RW (1997) A clinically based classification system for alcoholic chronic pancreatitis: summary of an inter-national workshop on chronic pancreatitis. Pancreas 14:215–221

Ammann RW, Muellhaupt B (1999) The natural history of pain in alcoholic chronic pancreatitis. Gastroenterology 116:1132–1140

Beger HG, Schlosser W, Friess HM, Buchler MW (1999) Duodenum-preserving head resection in chronic pancreatitis changes the natural course of the disease: a single-center 26-year experience. Ann Surg 230:512–519

Buchler MW, Friess H, Muller MW, et al. (1995) Randomized trial of duodenum-preserving pancreatic head resection versus pylorus-preserving Whipple in chronic pancreatitis. Am J Surg 169:65–69

Cahen DL, Gouma DJ, Yung Nio, et al. (2007) Endoscopic versus surgical drainage of the pancreatic duct in chronic pancreatitis. N Engl J Med 356:676–684

Di Sebastiano P, di Mola FF, Bockman DE, et al. (2003) Chronic pancreatitis: the perspective of pain generation by neuroimmune interaction. Gut 52:907–911

Frey CF, Smith GJ (1987) Description and rationale of a new operation for chronic pancreatitis. Pancreas 2:701–707

Gloor B, Friess H, Uhl W, Buchler MW (2001) A modified technique of the Beger and Frey procedure in patients with chronic pancreatitis. Dig Surg 18:21–25

Kahl S, Zimmermann S, Genz I, et al. (2003) Risk factors for failure of endoscopic stenting of biliary strictures in chronic pancreatitis: a prospective follow-up study. Am J Gastroenterol 98:2448–2453

Klempa I, Spatny M, Menzel J, et al. (1995) Pancreatic function and quality of life after resection of the head of the pancreas in chronic pancreatitis. A prospective, randomized comparative study after duodenum preserving resection of the head of the pancreas versus Whipple's operation. Chirurg 66:350–359

Traverso LW, Kozarek RA (1997) Pancreatoduodenectomy for chronic pancreatitis: anatomic selection criteria and subsequent long-term outcome analysis. Ann Surg 226:429–435

Witzigmann H, Max D, Uhlmann D, et al. (2003) Outcome after duodenum-preserving pancreatic head resection is improved compared with classic Whipple procedure in the treatment of chronic pancreatitis. Surgery 134:53–62

# 4
# Pancreas Divisum

**Andrew L. Warshaw**

## Pearls and Pitfalls

- Pancreas divisum refers to a congenital non-union of the dorsal and ventral pancreatic ducts. Classic pancreas divisum is found in 5% of Western populations.
- The functional implication of pancreas divisum is that secretions from the dorsal and ventral pancreatic segments must egress through separate orifices (the accessory or minor papilla and the major ampulla, respectively).
- Other anatomic variants in which the ventral duct may be entirely absent or in which the communication may be so narrow as to be functionally inadequate result in similar dependence on the accessory papilla route. These in aggregate account for up to 10–15% of the population.
- A more inclusive and utilitarian designation for the three anatomic groups, rather than pancreas divisum, is *dominant dorsal duct*, which indicates that the predominance of pancreatic secretions must flow through the accessory papilla.
- Pancreas divisum, or a dominant dorsal duct, leads to symptoms only if the accessory papilla is functionally or mechanically too narrow to allow unimpeded flow.
- Dominant dorsal duct anatomy combined with accessory papilla stenosis can lead to ductal hypertension, recurrent acute pancreatitis, "pancreatic pain", and rarely chronic obstructive pancreatitis.

K.I. Bland et al. (eds.), *Surgery of the Pancreas and Spleen*, DOI: 10.1007/978-1-84996-369-5_4, © Springer-Verlag London Limited 2011

- The diagnosis of pancreas divisum or other dominant dorsal duct configurations is made by pancreatography – either ERCP or MRCP. Despite functional or mechanical orificial stenosis, the diameter of the dorsal duct is usually normal.
- Direct evaluation of the size of the accessory papilla orifice and endoscopic manometry have been unreliable. US, EUS, and MRCP after secretin stimulation may demonstrate prolonged ductal dilation indicative of impaired emptying.
- Treatment is directed at the stenosis of the accessory papilla by endoscopic sphincterotomy or operative sphincteroplasty.
- Evidence of chronic pancreatitis, either at original presentation or after failed sphincter ablation, may require pancreaticoduodenectomy or lateral pancreatic duct drainage.

## Background and Significance

Pancreas divisum, classically the embryologic failure of fusion of the dorsal and ventral pancreatic anlage (segments), obligates that secretions from each portion have an independent outflow tract, depending heavily on the duct of Santorini and accessory papilla, rather than emptying via the duct of Wirsung and the ampulla of Vater, for all or most of the flow. A similar reliance on the dorsal duct and accessory papilla occurs if the connection between the two systems is filamentous and functionally stenotic (incomplete pancreas divisum) or if the ventral duct of Wirsung is absent (Fig. 4.1). In all, these variants are found in up to 20% of Western populations. The term "dominant dorsal duct" includes all three of these variants and is therefore preferable to the commonly used "pancreas divisum."

A dominant dorsal duct does not lead per se to clinical disease. Accessory papilla stenosis must coexist in order to cause ductal hypertension under conditions of augmented flow, as would occur during stimulation by meals (or challenge by exogenous secretin). This ductal "hypertension" is postulated

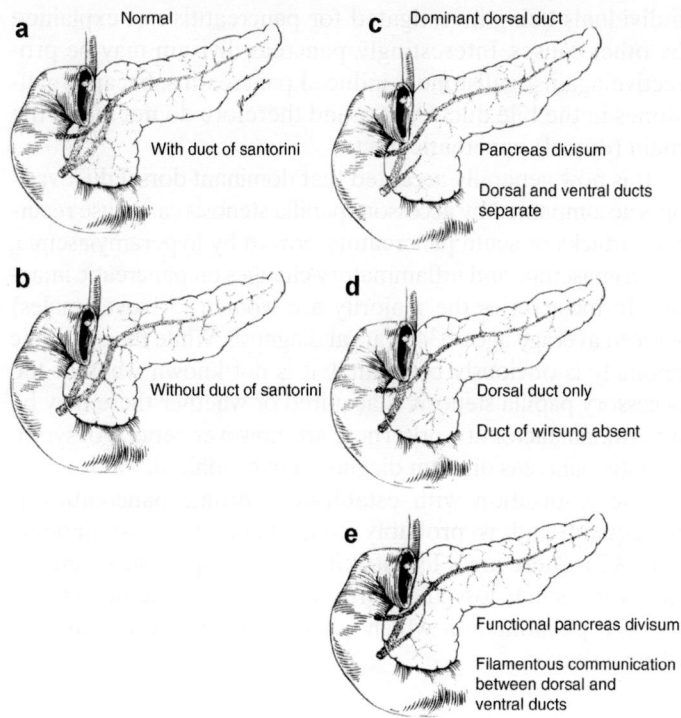

FIGURE 4.1. Variants of pancreatic duct anatomy which either allow for ventral orifice drainage or obligate dorsal drainage via the accessory papilla (including pancreas divisum).

to lead to recurrent acute pancreatitis, a pancreatic pain syndrome without other indicators of inflammation, or possibly chronic obstructive changes in pancreatic morphology.

## Clinical Presentation

Most individuals with dominant dorsal duct anatomy never develop clinical symptoms or sequelae. The anatomic variant may be discovered incidentally during pancreatography for other reasons but is significantly more common among individuals being investigated for pancreatitis not explained by other causes. Interestingly, pancreas divisum may be protective against gallstone – induced pancreatitis, because gallstones in the bile duct bypass, and therefore do not affect the main (dorsal) pancreatic duct.

It is now generally accepted that dominant dorsal duct variants accompanied by accessory papilla stenosis can cause recurrent attacks of acute pancreatitis, proven by hyperamylasemia, hyperlipasemia, and inflammatory changes on pancreatic imaging. In most series the majority are women (3:1 over males) with an average age of 34 years at diagnosis. While the anatomic anomaly is obviously congenital, it is not known whether the accessory papilla stenosis is acquired or whether there may be a hormonal factor at work. There are, however, reports of symptomatic pancreas divisum diagnosed in childhood.

The association with established chronic pancreatitis is infrequent and is probably coincidental in most patients (Fig. 4.2). There are a few striking and indisputable examples of severe acinar loss and fibrosis confined to the dorsal segment, a phenomenon which testifies to isolated dorsal duct obstruction.

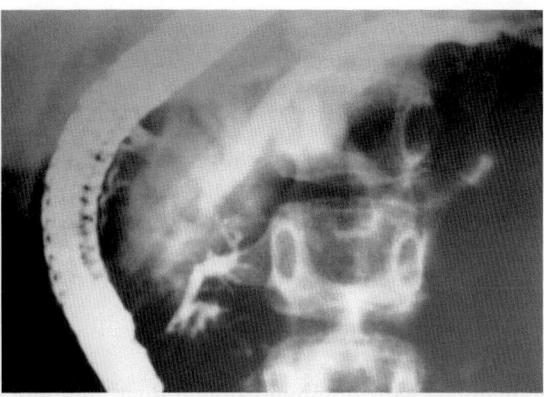

FIGURE 4.2. Pancreatogram showing chronic pancreatitis with a dilated main pancreatic duct in a patient with pancreas divisum. The ventral duct shows equal changes of chronic pancreatitis.

A syndrome of epigastric and back pain suggestive of a pancreatic origin, but without objective correlates of pancreatic inflammation, has also been attributed to pancreas divisum, albeit with greater skepticism. The inability to exclude unrelated pathology, including psychopathology, has led to a much higher rate of treatment failure.

Longitudinal observations often demonstrate infrequent attacks early on, perhaps only once every year or two, but with increasing frequency as the years go by. Similarly, pain may be sporadic at first but becomes daily and eventually continuous. Hyperamylasemia may occur early in the course but may cease later, thus obscuring the objective diagnosis.

The attacks of pancreatitis are almost universally mild. Complications of acute pancreatitis, such as necrosis and pseudocysts, are exceedingly rare. Similarly, the progression to diabetes and exocrine insufficiency has not been shown and should not be used as a rationale for pre-emptive treatment.

## Diagnosis

The diagnosis of dominant dorsal duct anatomy requires some form of direct pancreatography to delineate both the presence or absence of the ventral and dorsal ducts and the degree of communication between them. Magnetic resonance pancreatography (MRP) has improved such that accurate depiction of the duct system can often be obtained noninvasively (Fig. 4.3).

Typically the ventral duct in pancreas divisum extends only 2–4 cm from the major ampulla, short of the midline, and is formed from the confluence of fine, tapered branches servicing the caudal portion of the head and uncinate process (Fig. 4.4). This foreshortened ventral duct must not be confused with a ventral duct truncated by a neoplasm or by acquired obstruction from scarring in chronic pancreatitis or acute necrotizing pancreatitis. The morphology of acquired ventral duct obstruction, called false pancreas divisum, is

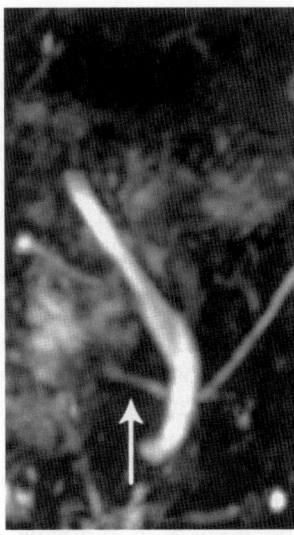

FIGURE 4.3. MR cholangiopancreatography demonstrating pancreatic duct anatomy in which the ventral duct is absent and the dorsal duct (arrow) serves the entire pancreas.

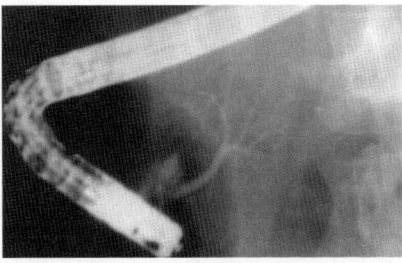

FIGURE 4.4. Endoscopic pancreatography via papilla of Vater; the pancreatic duct in the head of the gland is short and formed by the confluence of fine secondary branches.

differentiated easily from the congenital anomaly in that the visualized portion of the main ventral duct is broader, may be longer, and ends abruptly at the obstructing point, rather than tapering into its branched origins.

Inability to locate a ventral duct by ERCP should raise the suspicion of its absence and of the complete dependence on the dorsal duct and accessory papilla as the conduit for pancreatic exocrine secretins. Failure to appreciate this possibility will lead to a missed diagnosis. Cannulation of the accessory papilla (or MRP) will be necessary to confirm the anatomy (Fig. 4.5).

Visual estimation or sizing of the orifice of the accessory papilla by the endoscopist or surgeon has been unreliable, as has been the difficulty or ease of cannulation. Manometry through this tiny channel has had uncertain predictive value for selecting patients for either endoscopic or surgical treatment and has not been applied widely.

The dorsal duct, in the absence of true chronic pancreatitis, generally has a normal, non-dilated configuration even if the accessory papilla orifice is small. Significant persistent dilation has been present in only 3 of 200 pancreatograms in the author's experience and, when present, indicates chronic fibrotic changes. It should be recognized that pancreatography is most often performed while the subject is fasting, and pancreatic secretion is not being stimulated. If the accessory papilla is relatively stenotic, however, dilatation of the dorsal duct may occur after feeding (leading to ductal hypertension and sequelae). This circumstance can be reproduced by secretin administration (70 units intravenously).

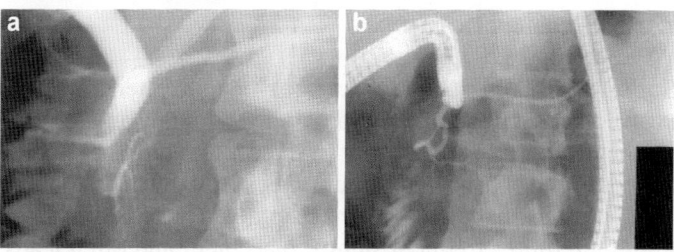

FIGURE 4.5. Endoscopic pancreatogram via the accessory papilla. (**a**) Classic pancreas divisum (the ventral duct has been opacified via a separate cannulation. (**b**) The dorsal duct system serves the entire pancreas (absent ventral duct system).

TABLE 4.1. Chance of beneficial outcome after accessory papilla sphincteroplasty.

| Ultrasound secretin text | Recurrent acute pancreatitis | Chronic pain only |
|---|---|---|
| Positive | 90% (19/21) | 94% (15/16) |
| Negative | 64% (7/11) | 21% (3/14) |

We described the use of ultrasonography during secretin stimulation to demonstrate delayed emptying of the dorsal duct suggestive of functional papillary stenosis. The characteristic finding of *prolonged* dorsal duct dilation (20–30 min), in contrast to the brief (1–3 min) dilation seen normally, has been reasonably predictive of a good treatment response to accessory papilla sphincterotomy or sphincteroplasty (Table 4.1). More recently, MRP and endoscopic ultrasonography (EUS) have been used in similar fashion to monitor dorsal duct responses to secretin.

It has been proposed that a therapeutic trial of accessory papilla stenting could predict which patients should benefit from enlarging the papillary orifice. There are insufficient data at present to reach a sound conclusion. It must be recognized also that much longer periods of stenting would be required if the attacks of pancreatitis or symptoms occur only infrequently.

# Endoscopic Therapy

Endoscopic approaches to accessory papilla stenosis have evolved from balloon dilatation alone to long-term stenting, sphincterotomy, and currently to the combination of sphincterotomy and short-term (about 2 weeks) stenting. Dilatation alone causes pancreatitis unacceptably often; long-term stenting requires frequent stent replacement and often leads to irreversible injury to the duct; sphincterotomy alone does not produce sufficient lasting benefit. Nonetheless, a randomized (unblinded) trial of long-term stenting by Lans and colleagues showed a 90% benefit (>50% reduction in pain, reduced emergency department visits and hospitalizations) versus 11% among control subjects over a mean follow-up of more than 2 years. That study at least lends support to the principle of treatment directed at relieving accessory papilla stenosis.

More recent investigations have reported successful use of a combination of sphincterotomy and short-term stenting. Lehman et al. reported a reduction in pain and days of hospitalization in 13 of 17 patients (76%) with recurrent acute pancreatitis, in 3 of 11 with chronic pancreatitis, and in 6 of 23 with a chronic pain syndrome. Even with short-term stenting, however, 50% of patients had changes in the dorsal duct at the time of stent removal. Kozarek and colleagues reported good results in 11 of 15 patients (73%) with recurrent acute pancreatitis, in 6 of 19 with chronic pancreatitis, and in only 1 of 5 with chronic pain; 20% of their patients had procedure or stent-related pancreatitis, and 12% had restenosis of the accessory papilla.

## Operative Therapy

The open operative approach to patients with symptoms related to a dominant dorsal duct and accessory papilla stenosis parallels that of endoscopic sphincterotomy and stenting but has the potential advantages of greater long-term patency and assured entry into the accessory papilla. The operation has been applied most successfully to symptomatic patients without changes of chronic pancreatitis (Table 4.2).

Operative enlargement of the orifice of the accessory papilla is accomplished by sutured sphincteroplasty through a transverse duodenotomy (Fig. 4.6). The accessory papilla is identified 2–3 cm proximal to the major papilla. If the gallbladder is to be removed, a catheter passed into the duodenum via the cystic duct will be helpful in placing the duodenotomy. The accessory papilla may be difficult to see among the duodenal folds and may be located most readily by gentle palpation on the medial duodenal wall. Secretin

TABLE 4.2. Outcomes of accessory papilla sphincteroplasty for dominant dorsal duct syndromes (pancreas divisum).

| | Total no. patients | Recurrent acute pancreatitis | | Chronic pain | | Restenosis % | Mean follow-up (months) |
|---|---|---|---|---|---|---|---|
| | | No. | % Success | No. | % Success | | |
| Warshaw (1990) | 88 | 43 | 82 | 45 | 56 | 7 | 53 |
| Madura (1986) | 30 | 11 | 82 | 19 | 77 | – | 31 |
| Keith (1989) | 21 | 13 | 100 | 8 | 75 | 5 | 53 |
| Bradley (1996) | 31 | 31 | 84 | – | – | 6 | 76 |

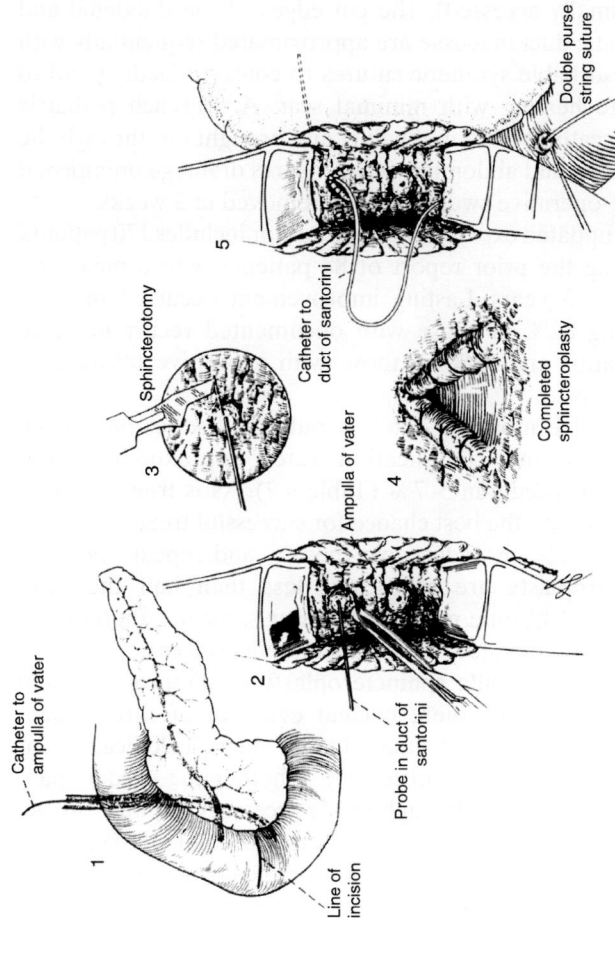

FIGURE 4.6. Technique of accessory papilla sphincteroplasty.

administration can be helpful in visualizing the miniscule orifice, which is then cannulated with a fine lachrymal duct probe. The anterosuperior lip of the papilla is incised over the probe, and the incision is extended between fine hemostatic clamps for about 1 cm (until the vestibule behind the papilla is maximally accessed). The cut edges of the duodenal and pancreatic duct mucosae are approximated sequentially with fine absorbable synthetic sutures to control bleeding and to promote healing with minimal scar. A 5-French pediatric feeding catheter, left in the duct and brought out through the duodenum and abdominal wall, ensures drainage unimpeded by post-operative swelling and is removed in 3 weeks.

The updated experience of the author includes 170 patients, mirroring the prior report of 88 patients, with a mean followup of 5 years. Lasting improvement occurred in 70%; including 82% of those with documented recurrent acute pancreatitis and 92% of those with a positive ultrasound-secretin test.

Operative mortality rates in published series have been under 1% and complication rates approximately 4%. Restenosis occurs in 5–7% (Table 4.2). As is true for endoscopic therapy, the best chance for successful treatment is the first one; salvage endoscopic therapy and repeat operative sphincteroplasty are efficacious less than half the time. Established fibrotic pancreatitis after sphincter therapy has failed may necessitate pancreaticoduodenectomy.

Accessory papilla sphincteroplasty is inappropriate and unsuccessful when there is clear evidence of chronic pancreatitis, including irregular dilated ducts, calcification, or exocrine/endocrine insufficiency. Whether the chronic pancreatitis was caused by high-grade accessory papilla obstruction or is a pathogenetically unrelated coincidence (i.e., 15% of patients with alcoholic or idiopathic chronic pancreatitis can be expected to have a dominant dorsal duct anatomy), the issue is moot and of no importance to the choice of therapy. Established chronic pancreatitis and its complications in patients with pancreas divisum are treated like those of any causation: side-to-side pancreaticojejunostomy (modified Puestow procedure), pancreaticoduodenectomy (Whipple procedure or its pylorus-preserving modification), or duodenum-sparing pancreatic head resection (Beger or Frey procedures) as the situation or surgeon's preference dictate.

As pancreas divisum becomes recognized more widely in childhood, the evolving principles of treatment remain the same as in adults. There are also case reports of isolated ventral pancreatitis in patients with pancreas divisum. The pathogenesis of this condition is obscure, but successful relief of pain has been achieved after either sphincteroplasty of the major ampulla and pancreatolithotomy or by pancreaticoduodenectomy.

## Selected Readings

Catalano MF, Lahoti S, Alcocer E, et al. (1998) Dynamic imaging of the pancreas using real-time endoscopic ultrasonography with secretin stimulation. Gastrointest Endosc 48:580

Kozarek RA, Ball TJ, Patterson DJ, et al. (1995) Endoscopic therapy in patients with pancreas divisum. Dig Dis Sci 40:1974

Lans JI, Geenen JE, Johanson JF, Hogan WJ (1992) Endo-scopic therapy in patients with pancreas divisum and acute pancreatitis: a prospective, randomized, controlled clinical trial. Gastrointest Endosc 38:430

Lehman CA, Sherman S, Nisi R, Hawes RH (1993) Pancreas divisum: Results of minor papilla sphincterotomy. Gastrointest Endosc 39:1

Neblett WW III, O'Neill JA Jr (2000) Surgical management of recurrent pancreatitis in children with pancreas divisum. Ann Surg 231:899

Warshaw AL, Simeone J, Schapiro RH, et al. (1985) Objective evaluation of ampullary stenosis with ultrasonography and pancreatic stimulation. Am J Surg 149:65–72

Warshaw AL, Simeone JF, Schapiro RH, Flavin-Warshaw B (1990) Evaluation and treatment of the dominant dorsal duct syndrome (pancreas divisum redefined). Am J Surg 159:59

# 5
# Pancreatic Pseudocysts

Åke Andrén-Sandberg

## Pearls and Pitfalls

- The terms *acute* and *chronic pseudocysts* are important clinically; the term acute usually refers to the association with *acute pancreatitis* and chronic to the association with *chronic pancreatitis*.
- Chronic pseudocysts most often are small, multiple, and of different sizes.
- Large pseudocysts(>20 cm) are usually only seen with acute pancreatitis.
- In children, trauma is the principal cause of pseudocysts; most resolve without treatment.
- Most pseudocysts that occur after an episode of acute pancreatitis resolve within 6 or 12 weeks.
- Pseudocysts that result from chronic pancreatitis almost never resolve and seldom give symptoms (those of chronic pancreatitis initiate pain).
- The risk of conservative treatment is minimal; serious complications, such as perforation, bleeding, infection, or gastrointestinal or biliary obstruction, are ≤10%.
- Errant diagnosis of the neoplastic "pseudocyst" is possible and usually occurs in the absence of a documented history of acute or chronic pancreatitis and when the lesion is small.

K.I. Bland et al. (eds.), *Surgery of the Pancreas and Spleen*, DOI: 10.1007/978-1-84996-369-5_5,
© Springer-Verlag London Limited 2011

- If the patient requires treatment for symptoms, percutaneous or endoscopic procedures are the approaches of choice; the choice of procedure depends on operator expertise.
- Open surgery is used less frequently today but remains an option if no other treatment modalities are available.
- Laparoscopic surgery is not superior to open surgery.

# Definitions

A pseudocyst presents as a cystic cavity adherent to the pancreas by inflammatory tissue. Typically, the wall of a pancreatic pseudocyst lacks an epithelial lining, and the cyst contains pancreatic secretions rich in amylase. These findings comprise the histopathologic components of the pancreatic pseudocyst. Historically, there have been several different clinical definitions of pancreatic pseudocysts – and there are probably more to come in the future. Today most clinically oriented definitions differentiate between acute peripancreatic fluid collections, pseudocysts, and pancreatic abscess. The majority of current literature addressing the stages of pseudocyst formation is consistent with the Atlanta classification system for acute pancreatitis. The more detailed descriptions include:

- *Acute peripancreatic fluid collections* – collections of fluid, usually ill-defined, occur early in the course of acute pancreatitis; located in or near the pancreas and lacking a wall of granulation or fibrous tissue.
- *Acute pseudocysts* – a collection of pancreatic secretions enclosed by a pseudocapsule of fibrous or granulation tissue and arising as a consequence of acute pancreatitis or pancreatic trauma; communication with the pancreatic ductal system is common(Fig. 5.1).
- *Chronic pseudocysts* – a collection of pancreatic secretions enclosed by a wall of fibrous or granulation tissue, arising as a consequence of chronic pancreatitis without an antecedent episode of acute pancreatitis; most, but not all, communicate with the pancreatic ductal system.

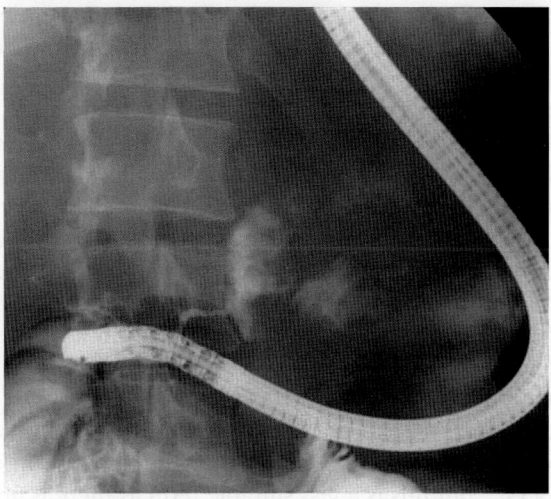

FIGURE 5.1. Endoscopic retrograde pancreatography (ERP) demonstrating a pseudocyst with connection to the pancreatic main duct.

- *Pancreatic abscess* – a circumscribed intra-abdominal collection of pus, usually in proximity with the pancreas, containing little or no pancreatic necrosis. This abscess arises as the consequence of acute pancreatitis, trauma, chronic pancreatitis, or after pancreatic invasive procedures.

Description of the separate entity of acute fluid collections in the Atlanta classification is important, because it documents the genesis for the development of acute pseudocysts and abscesses. Distinction between pseudocysts and acute fluid collections leads to a better understanding of the natural history of peripancreatic fluid collections and facilitates the treatment of these two separate entities, even though they represent a by-product of the same pathologic process. The presence of a well-defined wall composed of granulation or fibrous tissue and the communication with the pancreatic ductal system distinguishes the pseudocyst from an acute fluid collection. The pseudocyst is usually rich in pancreatic enzymes and is most often sterile. The formation and maturation of a pseudocyst usually requires 4 or more weeks (some clinicians state 6 weeks) from the onset of acute pancreatitis.

The differentiation in the Atlanta classification between acute and chronic pseudocyst formation is important but invites confusion. In the classification, the terms "acute" and "chronic" refer to the inflammatory process behind the pseudocyst, rather than to the mode of development or the symptomatology of the pseudocyst itself. This definition implies that an acute pseudocyst may have been known for months, whereas a chronic pseudocyst has been documented only recently (1–2 weeks). A further clue to the classification is that chronic pseudocysts are usually small, multiple, and of variable size.

Bacteria may be present in cultures of the pseudocyst. On occasion, the pancreatic pseudocyst is termed an "infected pseudocyst," but this is a less suitable term as there is no precise definition. Moreover, it is improbable from a biologic point of view to distinguish between the infected fluid collections and an abscess. Parenthetically, most positive cultures from pseudocysts without clinical indication of infection result from contamination that occurs during the culture procedure. When purulence is evident, the lesion is of course more correctly termed a "pancreatic abscess," at least by the Atlanta classification. (This usage of the term "pancreatic abscess" differs from past use of the term to describe infected necrosis complicating necrotizing pancreatitis and has been a point of contention among pancreatologists.) The relationship between acute fluid collections, pseudocysts, bacterial contamination, and confirmed bacterial infection of clinical significance is often difficult to differentiate. Many would prefer, therefore, that the term "infected pseudocyst" be discarded.

## Natural History

The widespread application of ultrasonography and computed tomography (CT) has advanced biomedical knowledge of the natural history of pancreatic pseudocysts. With resolution of the pseudocyst which may occur within a short period, it is improbable that free intraperitoneal rupture has occurred in the absence of peritoneal signs with the development of ascites. Theoretically, drainage into pancreatic lymphatics or the extrapancreatic retroperitoneal tissues may occur, as may internal drainage through the pancreatic ductal system after resolution of temporary obstruction of the duct.

For acute pseudocysts, the rate for spontaneous resolution is high. Because many patients diagnosed with acute pseudocysts will actually have *acute* fluid collections, the higher resolution rate will be evident. The recent prospective cohort study of a nonalcoholic population with acute pancreatitis revealed that 65% of "acute pancreatic pseudocysts" resolved spontaneously; this resolution typically occurs within 1 year. The size of the cyst does not appear to affect the probability of resolution, but *spontaneous resolution* is less probable if the pseudocyst has been present for a long duration after acute pancreatitis. Some authors contend that pseudocysts that are present at 12 weeks are unlikely to resolve spontaneously. Patients with pancreatic calcifications or other evidence of chronic pancreatitis have a low probability of spontaneous resolution of their pancreatic pseudocyst.

## Risk for Complications in Untreated Pancreatic Pseudocysts

In several early series in the 1970s, the incidence of complications in acute pseudocysts correlated directly with the duration of time the pseudocyst was present. In an early ultrasonographic study of acute pancreatitis, 20% of patients with early pseudocyst(<6 weeks) had a complication versus 46% with cysts that were 7–12 weeks old. Complications were evident in 75% of those with cysts beyond 13 weeks. Severe, possibly life-threatening complications in this group include intracystic hemorrhage, free perforation into the peritoneal cavity ("pancreatic ascites"), cyst infection (abscess), and fistula formation. These series probably included many patients with "fluid" collections secondary to necrotizing pancreatitis that were not, in retrospect, pancreatic pseudocysts. Pseudocysts may also be the genesis of recurrent pancreatitis that occurs secondary to outflow obstruction. The most severe complication, however, is bleeding during operative intervention for symptomatic pseudocysts.

More recent studies, however, have shown that in the absence of necrotizing pancreatitis, asymptomatic pancreatic pseudocysts have a much lower incidence($\leq 10\%$) of such serious complications.

Chronic pseudocysts almost never give rise to a life-threatening complication, probably because they are small and surrounded by harder, less vascular fibrous tissues. The complications seen result from external compression of the bile duct or intestinal tract (e.g., duodenum); in contrast, the pain experienced in these patients usually results from chronic pancreatitis rather than the resulting pseudocyst.

Compression of bile ducts by pseudocysts represents a special problem. In the patient with pancreatitis and evidence of biliary obstruction (increases in serum bilirubin and/or alkaline phosphatase), decompression of the obstructed biliary system should be performed (endoscopically, radiographically, or surgically) unless there is rapid, spontaneous abatement of the pseudocyst volume to allow decompression. Drainage of the pancreatic pseudocyst with bilioenteric anastomosis may avoid complications. It is important to determine objectively whether a creation of an operative bilioenteric diversion is necessary such that it can be accomplished synchronously with drainage of the pseudocyst. Because chronic pancreatitis is often a progressive disease, patients with cholestasis treated only with drainage of the pseudocyst should be followed closely for subsequent evidence of bile duct obstruction secondary to pancreatic fibrosis; the latter presentation will require bilioenteric diversion. Thoracic manifestations of pancreatic pseudocysts may occur and include mediastinal pseudocysts, pancreaticopleural fistulas with chronic pleural effusions, and the rare pancreaticobronchial fistulas and pancreaticopericardial fistulas with chronic pericardial effusions.

# Children

Pancreatic pseudocysts in children in the 5-to 10-year-old age group result most commonly with trauma. In a series of 48 patients, pancreatitis was caused by trauma or congenital anomalies in every child under 4 years of age; in contrast, in the child under 2 years, significant trauma is a less common etiology, and congenital causes predominate. In children with congenital causes, recurrent obstruction of the pancreatic duct may occur, giving rise to repeated attacks of pancreatitis with progressive tissue destruction.

Spontaneous resolution may occur in a significant number of documented pancreatic pseudocysts of children (e.g., 50% of trauma cases). Every major pancreatic trauma does not progress to pseudocyst; thus, conservative management is proposed for pancreatic trauma without ductal injuries.

## *Indications for and Options for Intervention*

The basic indications for pseudocyst drainage, whether performed by radiologic, endoscopic, or surgical measures, remain unchanged (Table 5.1). Symptomatic pseudocysts, infected pseudocysts (i.e., pancreatic abscesses), and enlarging pseudocysts that influence the function of adjacent organs require drainage. The necessity to drain a documented pseudocyst based on criteria of size alone must be questioned. Past recommendations that all large pseudocysts – usually defined as larger than 6 cm in diameter – should be drained once their wall has "matured" is anecdotal; rather, drainage is determined by the necessity to decompress its contents based on compression of contiguous organs with subsequent clinically progressive symptoms.

TABLE 5.1.  Proposed guidelines for pancreatic pseudocyst treatment.

Be certain that the pseudocyst is not a neoplastic cyst (if there is no acute or chronic pancreatitis documented, raise the suspicion level)

If possible, allow the pseudocyst time to mature (about 6 weeks)

Identify and address pseudoaneurysms

Evaluate for the presence of portal hypertension and gastric varices

Be certain that the pseudocyst is in close apposition to the gastric or duodenal wall

Optional: perform pancreatography by ERCP or MRCP to examine if there is a communication to duct

Use a familiar method of treatment:

- Percutaneous technique
- Endoscopic technique
- Surgical drainage
- Resection

## Operative Therapy

Operative intervention remains the standard for drainage of pseudocysts against which new methods have been compared –but this approach must now be questioned seriously as few open procedures are required due to the success of endoscopic drainage (Fig. 5.2). Surgical operations usually consist of open or laparoscopic gastrocystostomy, duodenocystostomy, Roux-en-Y-jejunocystostomy, or resection (e.g., tail resections). These operative procedures carry a 10–30% morbidity rate, a 1–5% mortality rate, and a 10–20% rate of recurrence; endoscopic drainage and percutaneous techniques compare favorably with the surgical "standard" and probably should be favored over open operative drainage whenever possible.

The necessity for operative drainage/resection is also predicated on whether the lesion is a pseudocyst or neoplastic cyst. Neoplastic cysts usually have a good prognosis even if the epithelial components of the cyst are malignant; these lesions

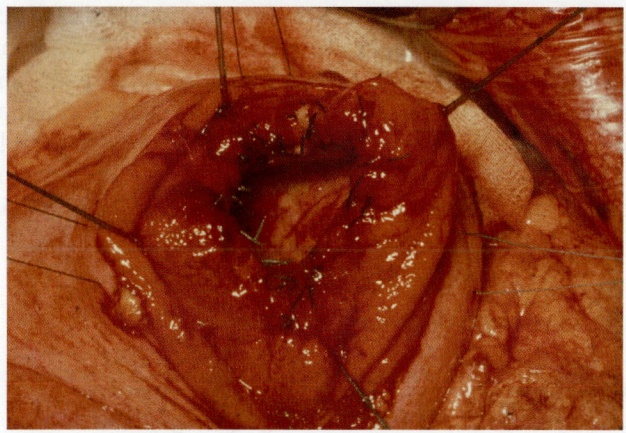

FIGURE 5.2. Surgical internal drainage of a pseudocyst: the pseudocyst is opened and anastomosed to a Roux limb of jejunum.

usually can be resected radically. Moreover, neoplastic cysts are more commonly diagnosed in earlier stages than adenocarcinoma. All "pseudocysts" should be treated as neoplasms when they occur in the absence of acute or chronic pancreatitis or trauma and if the lesion is small(<6cm). In these presentations, the patients should be referred to the specialist with a presumptive diagnosis of cystic pancreatic neoplasm. The "wait-and-see policy" should be abandoned, because the majority of presentations require resection, especially if the patient is younger, and the lesion is localized to the pancreatic tail.

No evidence exists that laparoscopic interventions are superior to open surgery for pancreatic pseudocysts. Laparoscopy *can* be used, but it is recommended only if the surgeon is well familiarize with both laparoscopy and open pancreatic surgery.

## Non-surgical Interventions

At present at least two forms of active therapy of pancreatic pseudocysts are available: percutaneous drainage and endoscopic drainage, and combinations of the same. Controversy exists concerning which of these techniques should be offered to the patient with initial therapy. Endoscopic ultrasonography(EUS) may assist drainage localization and may decrease the risks associated with the procedure. Resolution rates after surgical and nonsurgical methods are comparable, but clinical and technical aspects may mandate one method over the other. Each patient will require an individual, multidisciplinary approach to ensure optimal treatment outcomes.

## Percutaneous Treatment

Percutaneous catheter drainage of symptomatic pancreatic pseudocysts under CT or ultrasonographic guidance is a valuable adjunct of pseudocyst management. Diagnostic percutaneous aspiration of peripancreatic collection can be performed readily, but simple needle aspiration alone is an ineffective therapy (except as a temporary measure). Insertion of a pigtail catheter allows the cyst to remain collapsed, and 60–80% of pseudocysts may be drained successfully in this manner.

The current practice indications for percutaneous treatment of pseudocysts are essentially identical to those for surgical treatment. The percutaneous technique may be especially useful in the management of the immature symptomatic pseudocyst; moreover, this type of drainage can be performed in all patients, including those at high risk. Contraindications to percutaneous drainage of pseudocysts include:

- Collections associated with a solid or non-drainable pancreatic mass or with subtotal glandular necrosis (more than 50% parenchymal necrosis)
- Suspicion of malignancy
- Lack of a safe access route
- Recent or active hemorrhage into the collection
- Presence of a documented pseudoaneurysm
- Collections associated with obstruction of the main pancreatic duct (especially with a complete cut-off of the pancreatic duct proximal to the region of the pseudocyst)

## Endoscopic Treatment

The crucial anatomic feature that defines the potential for endoscopic drainage of a pseudocyst is that it lies in close association(within1cm)with the stomach or duodenum. The wall of the stomach or the duodenum is a common boundary of the pseudocyst between which the thick inflammatory peel forms a poorly defined interface. This association allows an enterostomy to be performed without concern for leakage into a potential space between the pseudocyst wall and the stomach and duodenum, which could develop if the pseudocyst and digestive walls were not in close apposition.

Pancreatic stenting is used to treat pancreatic duct strictures and ductal hypertension and may provide considerable improvement of pain. Thus, the technique is well-described and practiced internationally. In addition, the pancreatic duct may be stented by the transpapillary route or the pseudocyst cavity itself drained directly via a transpapillary stent. The long-term efficacy of pancreatic ductal stenting is still not well-defined.

Endoscopic transmural drainage should be considered only if the wall of the pseudocyst is in close apposition to the gastric or duodenal wall; endoscopic visualization of a bulge caused by intraluminal pressure guides the operators endoscopically created entry site into the pseudocyst. Pancreatography, magnetic resonance cholangiopancreatography (MRCP), or endoscopic retrograde cholangiopancreatography (ERCP) may assist visualization before any attempt at drainage is made. Whenever possible, anatomic abnormalities, such as distal strictures, duct disruptions, or pancreatic duct stones, should be addressed by endoscopic techniques to ensure long-term success. The performance of endoscopic pancreatography also permits the endoscopist to assess the feasibility of transpapillary drainage. Transpapillary drainage should be preferred to alternative methods for drainage, because this technique carries the least morbidity.

Bleeding during endoscopic drainage may be severe, because there are very few means to control major hemorrhage nonsurgically. Therefore, while endoscopy is a valuable tool in treating pseudocysts, the existence of a pseudoaneurysm is a distinct contraindication to endoscopic drainage in all patients; the presence of portal hypertension with gastric or duodenal varices is a strong relative contraindication.

## Precautions for Treatment

Irrespective of the planned technical approach for treatment of acute pseudocysts, the surgeon should allow the pseudocyst time to mature. The pseudocyst with a mature wall allows a simpler and more predictable outcome; further, the end result is a decreased risk of recurrence.

On occasion, a pseudoaneurysm is mistaken for a pseudocyst; usually pseudoaneurysms are rather small and with modern radiologic techniques (dynamic multislice CT with or without ultrasonography) are identified preoperatively. It is essential that identification of the pseudoaneurysm be determined early in the planned treatment to avoid exsanguinating hemorrhage.

For patients with chronic pancreatitis, the surgeon should also evaluate for the possible presence of portal hypertension and gastric varices before treatment to avoid major hemorrhagic events.

## Selected Readings

Andrén-Sandberg Å, Dervenis C (2004) Pancreatic pseudocysts in the 21st century. Part I: classification, pathophysiology, ananatomic considerations and treatment. JPancreas (Online) 5:8–24

Andrén-Sandberg Å, Dervenis C (2004) (2004) Pancreatic pseudocysts in the 21st century. Part II: natural history. J Pancreas (Online) 5:65–70

Byrne MF, Mitchell RM, Baillie J (2002) Pancreatic pseudo-cysts. Curr Treat Options Gastroenterol 5:331–338

Nealon WH, Walser E (2005) Surgical management of com-plications associated with percutaneous and/or endoscopic management of pseudocyst of the pancreas. Ann Surg 241:948–957

Pitchumoni CS, Agarwal N (1999) Pancreatic pseudocysts. When and how should drainage be performed? Gastroenterol Clin North Am 23:615–639

Sharma SS, Bhargawa N, Govil A (2002) Endoscopic management of pancreatic pseudocyst: a long-term follow-up. Endoscopy 34:203–207

Singhal D, Kakodkar R, Sud R, Chaudhary A (2006) Issues in management of pancreatic pseudocysts. JOP.JPancreas (Online) 7:502–507

Vitas GJ, Sarr MG (1992) Selected management of pancreatic pseudocysts: operative versus expectant management. Surgery 111:123–130

Vosoghi M, Sial S, Garrett B, et al. (2002) EUS-guided pancreatic pseudocyst drainage: review and experience at Harbor-UCLA Medical Center. MedGenMed 4:2–5

# 6

# Obstructive Jaundice: Preoperative Evaluation

Juan Pekolj and Martín Palavecino

## Pearls and Pitfalls

- The most common cause of obstructive jaundice is choledocholithiasis.
- Malignant neoplasms should be suspected in older patients (> 50 years old) presenting with painless jaundice.
- In newborn patients, biliary atresia must be suspected.
- Serum tumor markers are not sensitive or specific for malignancy in patients with obstructive jaundice. They should not be used as the sole diagnostic test.
- Ultrasonography (US) is an inexpensive and useful diagnostic tool in jaundiced patients.
- Endoscopic Retrograde Cholangiopancreatography (ERCP) or Percutaneous Transhepatic Cholangiography (PTC) may be necessary for preoperative planning or eventually treatment.
- Magnetic Resonance Cholangiopancreatography (MRCP) is a useful tool to determine the level of biliary obstruction and may obviate the need for invasive imaging.
- Jaundice after cholecystectomy should prompt evaluation for choledocholithiasis or bile duct injury.

K.I. Bland et al. (eds.), *Surgery of the Pancreas and Spleen*, DOI: 10.1007/978-1-84996-369-5_6,
© Springer-Verlag London Limited 2011

# Introduction

Obstructive jaundice is a common condition prompting surgical consultation. Over the past two decades, advances in imaging, endoscopy, and surgical technique have allowed a precise diagnosis and optimal management of patients with obstructive jaundice. Despite these advances in technology, the clinical history remains an important part during the evaluation (Table 6.1).

# Clinical Evaluation

The surgeon should evaluate a jaundiced patient according to the following questions:

1. *Is the jaundice related to an obstructive or non-obstructive process?*
   The surgeon should obtain information about previous episodes of jaundice, liver disease, and risk factors for hepatotoxicity and gallstones. The diagnosis possibilities can be narrowed considerably with adequate clinical assessment. The presence of fever, chills, and right upper quadrant pain (Charcot's triad) suggests cholangitis due to biliary obstruction. If the symptoms are acute, the surgeon should suspect a benign pathology. Patients who present with progressive anorexia, weight loss, deterioration of the performance status and/or vague abdominal complaints should prompt suspicion of a malignant etiology.

TABLE 6.1. Evaluation of the jaundiced patient

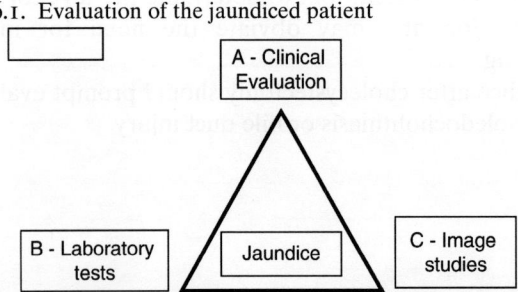

2. *Is biliary obstruction present, is it in the proximal, mid, or distal bile duct?*
   A palpable gallbladder may suggest the obstruction is below the cystic duct insertion in the bile duct. Imaging is necessary to definitively localize the site of biliary obstruction.

3. *Is the obstruction secondary to a stone or stenosis?*
   Choledocholithiasis is a common cause of obstructive jaundice and can be suspected by a careful, thorough history and confirmed with diagnostic imaging. When a patient develops jaundice in the immediate postoperative period after a cholecystectomy, residual choledocholithiasis or bile duct injury must be considered and evaluated.

4. *Is the obstruction secondary to a benign or malignant condition?*
   A complete clinical evaluation is necessary to differentiate between benign or malignant etiologies. In the absence of a previous biliary procedure, benign strictures are uncommon. Benign strictures due to primary sclerosing cholangitis may be suspected in patients with a history of ulcerative colitis.

## Laboratory Tests

The main objective of laboratory tests is to determine whether the jaundice is related to an obstructive or non-obstructive cause. The basic serum tests that should be obtained are:

- Total bilirubin/direct (conjugated) bilirubin
- AST/ALT
- Alkaline-phosphatase (ALP), 5'-nucleotidase (5NT), gamma-glutamyltransferase (GGT)

Jaundice is usually evident when the total bilirubin level exceeds 3 mg/dL. Hyperbilirubinemia may be caused by the un-conjugated (indirect bilirubin), conjugated (direct bilirubin) or both fractions. The indirect fraction can be increased in many non-obstructive disorders involving prehepatic and hepatic disorders (hemolysis, Gilbert's Syndrome, Crigler-Najjar's Syndrome, massive transfusion, etc.). Increase in the direct fraction may be secondary to biliary obstruction or non-obstructive disorders of hepatic clearance of bile, such as Rotor Syndrome, Dubin-Johnson Syndrome, hepatic granulomatosis, primary biliary cirrhosis, sarcoidosis, and tuberculosis.

Some diseases, such as acute viral hepatitis, toxic hepatitis (paracetamol poisoning, Amanita phalloides), alcoholic hepatitis, Budd-Chiari's Syndrome, Wilson's disease, hemochromatosis, and cirrhosis, can lead to increases in both fractions (mixed hyperbilirubinemia). As a general rule, AST and ALT levels are increased in primary hepatocellular diseases. However, moderate increases (twofold to threefold) of transaminases can be observed in biliary obstructions. In choledocholithiasis, AST and ALT may be increased before the serum bilirubin increases, but the AST and ALT typically normalize before bilirubin returns to normal. In contrast, obstructive jaundice leads to notable and dominant increases in the ALP, GGT, and 5NT levels. Serum albumin and prothrombin time (PT) are more accurate markers of liver function and are generally not useful in early jaundice. One exception might be the patient with a long history of jaundice. Prolonged extrahepatic obstruction may cause malabsorption of vitamin K with a subsequent coagulopathy (increased PT); similarly, chronic obstructive jaundice can lead to hepatocellular biliary cirrhosis with liver failure (decreased serum albumin) and cirrhosis.

Some laboratory tests are useful to determine specific diseases, such as copper levels in Wilson's disease, hepatitis antigens and antibodies in the viral hepatitis, and α-1 antitrypsin levels in α-1 antitrypsin deficiency.

Increased tumoral markers, such as CA19-9 (biliary and pancreatic neoplasms), CEA (metastasis from colorectal cancers, especially with lymph nodes in the porta hepatis), may occasionally be useful. However, normal levels of these markers do not exclude malignancy, and mild increased levels may be observed in benign conditions.

## Imaging Studies

Several methods of imaging have become available for evaluation of jaundiced patients and include (Table 6.2):

TABLE 6.2. Sensitivity, specificity, advantages, and disadvantages of each image study.

| Study | Sensitivity (%) | Specificity (%) | Advantages | Disadvantages |
|---|---|---|---|---|
| US/EUS | 55–91 | 82–95 | Non-invasive, portable, inexpensive | Obese patients and bowel gas may prevent adequate visualization, operator dependence |
| CT | 63–96 | 93–100 | Non-invasive, good resolution, no operator dependence | Intravenous contrast, more expensive |
| ERCP | 89–98 | 89–100 | Direct observation; allows biopsy and intervention | May require general anesthesia; risk of pancreatitis and duodenal perforation (~3%) |
| PTC | 98–100 | 89–100 | Direct observation, allows intervention | May require general anesthesia; difficult in non-dilated bile ducts |
| MRCP | 82–100 | 92–98 | Non-invasive | May cause apnea, claustrophobia; expensive |

- Transcutaneous ultrasonography (US)
- Endoscopic ultrasonography (EUS)
- Computed tomography (CT)
- Magnetic resonance cholangio pancreatography (MRCP)
- Endoscopic retrograde cholangio pancreatography (ERCP)
- Percutaneous transhepatic cholangiography

In general, the non-invasive modalities are used initially with the more invasive tests reserved for diagnostic uncertainty or for therapy.

## Ultrasonography

Ultrasonography is an excellent, non-invasive, and cost-effective modality utilized frequently as the initial diagnostic evaluation of the jaundiced patient. Intra-or extrahepatic biliary tract dilation, choledocholithiasis, gallbladder abnormalities, and occasionally pancreatic head abnormalities may be identified (Fig. 6.1). However, overlying bowel gas or large body habitus precludes adequate evaluation. Common bile

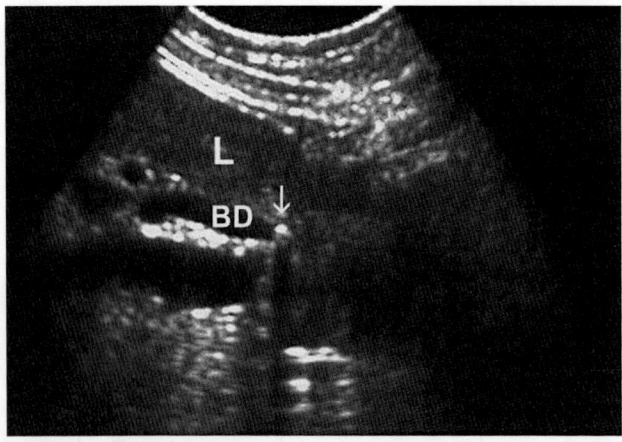

FIGURE 6.1. Ultrasonography showing a common bile duct stone.

duct can be mildly dilated (up to 8-10 mm) in cholecystecto-mized patients. With US, it is possible to determine (in 90% of patients) the level of obstruction in the bile ducts.

## Endoscopic Ultrasonography

Although more invasive, EUS has several advantages over transabdominal ultrasonography. EUS allows excellent evalua-tion of the biliary tract. EUS also avoids problems of overlying bowel gas and the obese body habitus that plagues transab-dominal ultrasonography. In periampullary tumors, EUS can accurately determine the level of tumoral invasion in the duo-denum. EUS can also evaluate regional lymph nodes and pro-vides the opportunity for transluminal fine needle aspiration biopsy. The primary limitation of EUS is that it depends on the endoscopist's experience; i.e., EUS is operator-dependent.

## Computed Tomography

Abdominal CT with intravenous contrast adds the ability to evaluate anatomy, assess local, regional, and distant abnor-malities and obviates the operator dependence of ultrasonog-raphy. CT allows identifying small lesions and it can localize the level of obstruction most of the time, although it is less sensitive than US in detecting choledocholithiasis, CT is invaluable when malignancy is suspected (Fig. 6.2).

## Magnetic Resonance Cholangio-Pancreatography

The property of static fluids to resonate in the T2 mode of MR allows excellent imaging of the biliary tract (and pan-creatic duct). With appropriate software, 3D reconstruc-tion is possible. The disadvantages of this method are the cost of the hardware, the unavailability of MR, and the

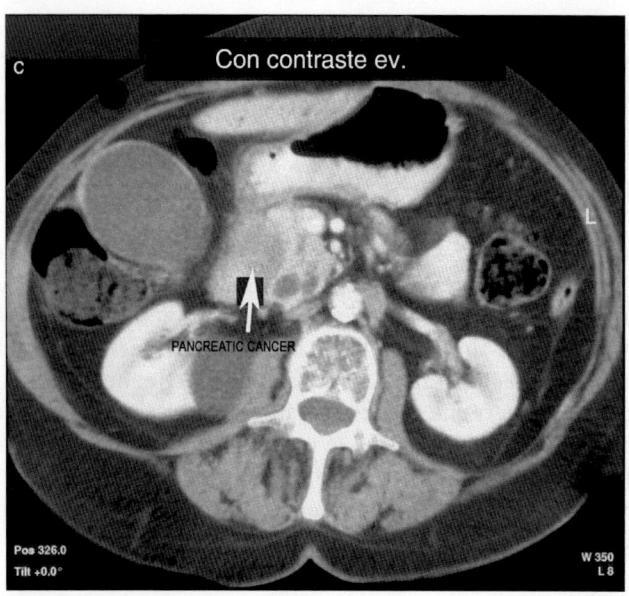

FIGURE 6.2.  CT showing a pancreatic head cancer, bile duct dilation, distended gallbladder.

necessity of general anesthesia in claustrophobic patients. MRCP is an excellent study to determine the cause and level of obstruction with a sensitivity of 95% and specificity of 94% (Fig. 6.3). In addition, MR will assess the tumoral anatomy, vascular involvement, and other parameters for staging.

## Endoscopic Retrograde Cholangio-Pancreatography

ERCP is an invasive method of direct ductal imaging. ERCP requires endoscopic insertion of a catheter through the ampulla of Vater with administration of intraductal

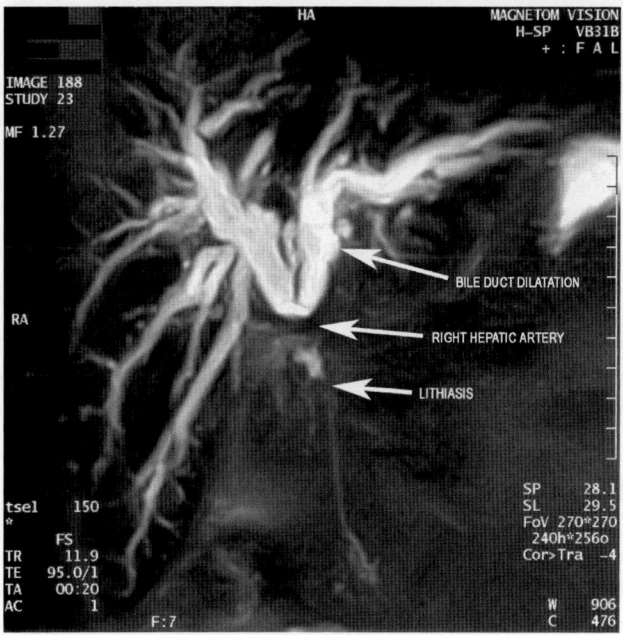

FIGURE 6.3. MRCP showing bile duct dilation secondary to a bile duct stone.

radiographic contrast; fluoroscopy provides excellent "direct'" cholangiography allowing precise delineation of choledo- cholithiasis, evidence of intraluminal masses, extraluminal compression, and level of obstruction. The ability to perform biopsy and brushings for cytology adds to the diagnostic abil- ity of this study. ERCP has the advantage over other diagnos- tic methods of allowing therapeutic intervention, such as clearance of choledocholithiasis and stenting of strictures when appropriate. Despite ERCP being a relatively safe pro- cedure, the overall complication rate is 3% and includes: pancreatitis, duodenal perforation, and bleeding after sphincterectomy.

# Percutaneous Transhepatic Cholangiography

Percutaneous transhepatic cholangiography (PTC) is performed by percutaneously placing a Chiba needle and transhepatically into a peripheral bile duct. Then using the Seldinger technique a catheter is inserted over a guide wire and direct cholangiography with fluoroscopy is obtained. PTC is a valuable technique in patients with complete biliary obstruction. PTC allows to delineate the anatomy above the level of obstruction, which may not be visible by ERCP. PTC also provides the opportunity to obtain brushings for cytology and palliate the obstruction by placing a drainage or stenting.

# Differential Diagnosis

The differential diagnosis of (surgical) mechanical obstructive jaundice can be categorized into causes of intrinsic obstruction (intraluminal or bile duct wall) or extrinsic compression from extraluminal/extramural etiologies (Table 6.3). A suggested diagnostic algorithm for the evaluation of obstructive jaundice is presented in Fig. 6.4.

TABLE 6.3.  Differential diagnosis of mechanical obstructive jaundice.

| Intrinsic obstruction | Extrinsic compression |
|---|---|
| Choledocholithiasis | Pancreatic head adenocarcinoma |
| Benign biliary strictures (e.g. primary sclerosing cholangitis) | Ampullary adenocarcinoma |
| | Chronic pancreatitis |
| Cholangiocarcinoma | Periductal adenopathy |
| Biliary atresia | Mirizzi Syndrome |
| Choledochal cysts | |

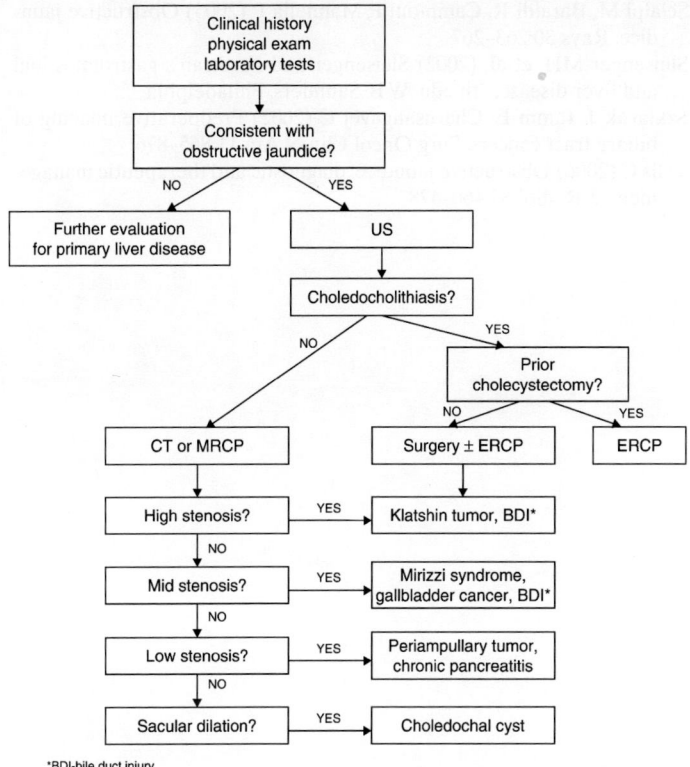

FIGURE 6.4. Diagnostic algorithm for the management of obstructive jaundice.

# Selected Reading

Kondo S, Isayama H, Akahane M, et al. (2005) Detection of common bile duct stones: comparison between endoscopic ultrasonography, magnetic resonance cholangiography, and helical-computed-tomographic cholangiography. Eur J Radiol 54:271–275

Pekolj J, Pietrani M, Mazza O, et al. (1999) MR cholangio-pancreatography for biliopancreatic pathologies. Rev Argen Cir 77:218–228

Scialpi M, Baraldi R, Campioni P, Mannella P (2005) Obstructive jaundice. Rays 30:263–267

Sleisenger MH, et al. (2002) Sleisenger and Fordtran's gastrointestinal and liver disease, 7th edn. W.B. Saunders, Philadelphia

Szklaruk J, Tamm E, Charnsangavej C (2002) Preoperative imaging of biliary tract cancers. Surg Oncol Clin N Am 11:865–876

Valls C (2006) Obstructive jaundice: diagnostic and therapeutic management. J Radiol 87:460–478

# 7
# Cystic Neoplasms of the Pancreas

**Michael G. Sarr and George H. Sakorafas**

## Pearls and Pitfalls

- Beware the cystic lesion in the pancreas in a patient without previous pancreatitis.
- The most common cystic neoplasms of the pancreas are:
  - Serous cystadenoma.
  - Mucinous cystic neoplasms (MCN).
  - Intraductal papillary mucinous neoplasms (IPMN).
- In the patient without a history of pancreatopathy, a cystic lesion in the pancreas is a cystic neoplasm until proven otherwise.
- In the older patient with idiopathic chronic pancreatitis (especially with a dilated duct), think IPMN.
- The most important point of differentiation in cystic neoplasms is whether the epithelium is serous or mucinous.
- Serous cystic neoplasms are benign.
- Mucinous cystic neoplasms are either overtly or potentially malignant.
- Ideally, all mucinous cystic lesions should be resected; lesions < 2 cm remain controversial.
- Biopsy of the wall of all "pseudocysts" is necessary before enteric drainage.
- Cystic neoplasms are best treated by anatomic resection.
- Resection of IPMN warrants frozen section of margins; if positive, then "creeping" resection is indicated.

K.I. Bland et al. (eds.), *Surgery of the Pancreas and Spleen*, DOI: 10.1007/978-1-84996-369-5_7, © Springer-Verlag London Limited 2011

- After resecting serous or non-invasive mucinous cystic neoplasms, surveillance imaging is not needed.
- After resecting invasive or non-invasive IPMN, surveillance is necessary with CT and/or endoscopic ultrasonography.
- Although used, adjuvant chemoradiation therapy for these malignant cystic lesions is of unproven benefit.

Advances in and access to non-invasive imaging, such as transabdominal ultrasonography(US), thin-section spiral computed tomography (CT), and magnetic resonance cholangiopancreatography (MRCP), have allowed us as physicians to visualize cystic lesions in the pancreas recognized only rarely in the past. Complicating this scenario is the recognition of such cystic lesions in asymptomatic patients, raising many questions about appropriate treatment of these newly appreciated cystic lesions of the pancreas.

Cystic lesions of the pancreas may be benign or malignant, neoplastic or non-neoplastic, congenital or acquired, or inflammatory or non-inflammatory, or may arise from adjacent tissues/organs actually outside the pancreas (Table 7.1). The first order of business in evaluation of these cystic lesions

TABLE 7.1. Most common cystic lesion of the pancreas.

| Neoplastic | Non-neoplastic |
|---|---|
| **Most common** | **Inflammatory** |
| Serous cystic neoplasm | Pseudocyst |
| Mucinous cystic neoplasm | Postnecrotic peripancreatic |
| Intraductal papillary mucinous neoplasm | Fluid collection |
|  | Echinococcal disease |
| **Rare** | **Congenital** |
| Cystic islet cell (neuroendocrine neoplasm) | Primary type pancreatic cyst |
| Solid pseudopapillary neoplasm | von Hippel Lindau disease |
| Lymphangioma | **Peripancreatic** |
|  | Left adrenal cysts |
|  | Retroperitoneal cysts |

is to determine whether the cystic lesion is neoplastic (cystic neoplasm) or non-neoplastic. *Beware* the patient with a cystic lesion in the pancreas who has no history of pancreatopathy (acute pancreatitis, chronic pancreatitis, trauma, etc.), because other benign, non-inflammatory cysts are very rare. *Cystic lesions in these patients should be considered as cystic neoplasms until proven otherwise.* Differentiation depends on history, imaging, and even sampling of intracystic fluid (see below – DIFFERENTIATION).

## Classification of Cystic Neoplasms

Cystic neoplasms include primary serous cystic neoplasms, primary mucinous cystic neoplasms, intraductal papillary mucinous cystic neoplasms, and the very rare cystic islet cell neoplasms, the solid pseudopapillary neoplasms that usually arise in young women, and ductal cancers with cystic necrosis.

### Serous Cystic Neoplasms

Serious cystic neoplasms (SCN) are routinely benign neoplasms, i.e. serous cystadenomas (although serous cystadeno-*carcinomas* have been reported, they are *exceedingly* rare). These SCNs are most common (75%) in older women (mean age 60–70 years), are often asymptomatic (>50%), arise throughout the gland, and cause symptoms by a mass effect – usually vague abdominal discomfort and not by obstructing the bile or pancreatic ducts. Systemic symptoms, such as weight loss, or obstructing symptoms, such as jaundice or gastric outlet obstruction, are very rare, because these are benign neoplasms. Their histology involves a single layer of serous, *non-mucinous* epithelium which lines multiple, small cystic areas (each individual cyst is almost always < 2 cm, and often microscopic) (Fig. 7.1a), thus, their old and now inappropriate name of "microcystic" adenomas. On gross examination, average tumor size is about 5 cm but can range from 2 to –20 cm; some serous cystadenomas appear to involve the entire gland. Cutting across the specimen shows multiple small cystic areas with a

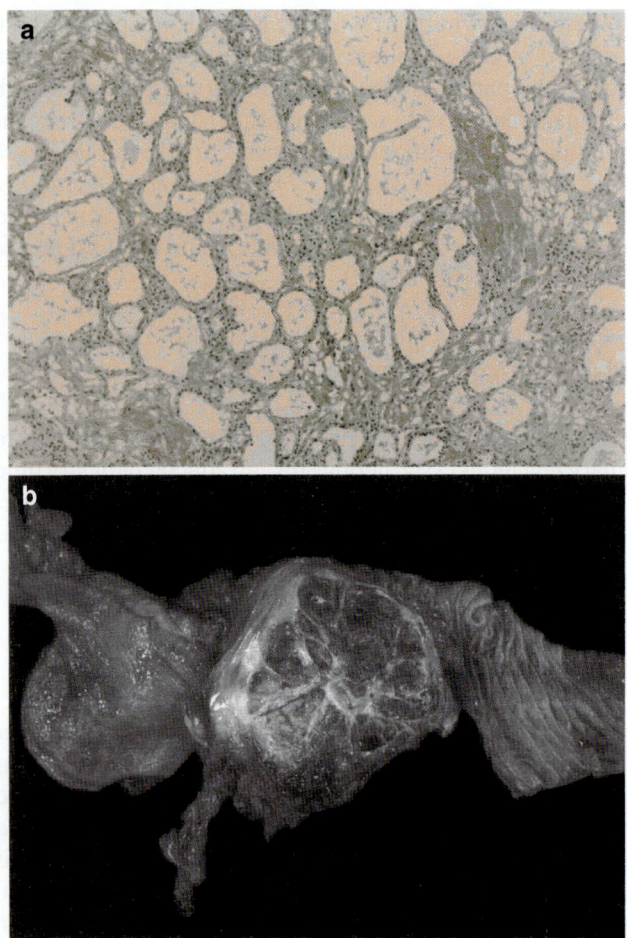

FIGURE 7.1. Common cystic neoplasms of the pancreas. (a) SCN –
note single layer of serous epithelium without dysplasia. (b) SCN –
note presence of multiple small cysts. (c) MCN – note the spectrum
of change within neoplasm showing benign mucinous epithelium
with other areas of dysplasia. (d) Note multiple large mucoid cysts.
(e) IPMN – note papillary changes with mucinous epithelium and
spectrum of dysplastic changes (a and b reprinted from Pykeetal.,
1992. With permission. (e) Reprinted from Loftus et al., 1996.
Copyright 1996. With permission from the American
Gastroenterological Association).

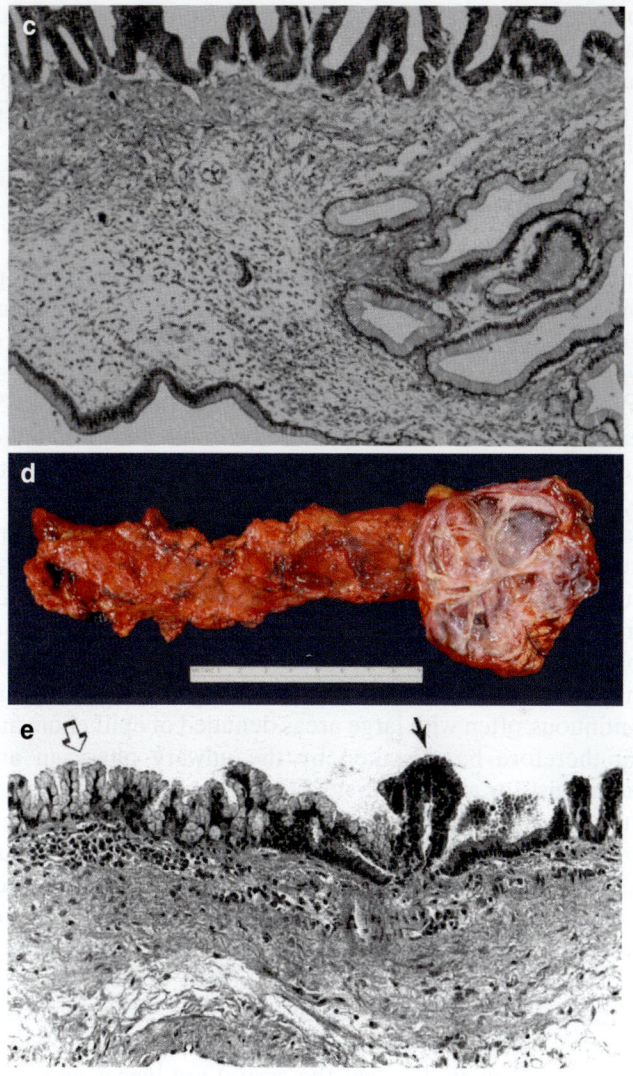

FIGURE 7.1. (continued).

honeycomb-like appearance; the cysts are composed of thin walls and contain a clear intracystic fluid. There is often central scarring and calcification (~30%) of the stroma with notably very little if any surrounding pancreatic inflammation (Fig. 7.1a, b).

## Mucinous Cystic Neoplasms

Unlike the SCNs, MCNs have a much different tumor biology and are either potentially malignant, contain pre-malignant *carcinoma-in-situ*, or less commonly (~10–15%) have areas of overtly malignant cells with tissue invasion. Virtually all patients (>95%) with MCN are women (mean age 40–50 years), and most all lesions tend to be in the body and tail of the gland. Many of the larger lesions are asymptomatic (>50%), but, when present, symptoms are usually from a mass effect; jaundice is rare, and constitutional symptoms, such as weight loss and anorexia, should raise suspicion of mucinous cystadeno*carcinoma*. These neoplasms contain larger cysts (each usually cyst > 2 cm) lined by a mucinous epithelium (Fig. 7.1c, d). However, the histopathology is unique for several reasons: (1) the lining is notoriously discontinuous, often with large areas denuded of epithelium and can therefore be mistaken by the unwary physician and pathologist for a pseudocyst; (2) the mucinous epithelium is often "proliferative" with areas of benign mucinous epithelium, while in other areas the cells can be atypical, heaped up, dysplastic, forming polypoid excrescences and frankly carcinomatous, either as *carcinoma-in situ* disease or with areas of tissue invasion, all within the same neoplasm – thus the designation as "proliferative" and potentially or overtly malignant; and (3) the stroma within the MCN has very characteristic histologic features of ovarian stroma, thus the marked predilection for women. Grossly, the cyst(s) are bigger and filled with a thicker, mucinous fluid. Septae or papillary epithelial changes are usually evident, and the peri-neoplastic parenchyma is almost always without reaction or scarring as occurs with inflammatory pancreatic pseudocysts; pericystic "reaction" may suggest an invasive focus – cystadenocarinoma.

## Intraductal Papillary Mucinous Neoplasms

This newly appreciated mucinous neoplasm with definite malignant potential, even more so than for the primary mucinous cystic neoplasms, arises from the pancreatic ducts. Unlike SCN and MCN, symptoms usually are present and consist of abdominal pain, steatorrhea, or weight loss. Clinically, the presentation may be similar to that of chronic pancreatitis with recurrent acute attacks or even a presentation of typical cancer of the pancreas. IPMN is a bit more common in men (60–70%) and is recognized usually in 60-to 75-year-old patients. The imaging procedures (see below) often show a dilated pancreatic duct and an atrophic pancreas, very suggestive of chronic pancreatitis; undoubtedly, many of these patients in the past were treated as idiopathic chronic pancreatitis and some later died of "mucinous ductal carcinoma". Histologically, the pancreatic ducts are lined with a mucinous, papillary epithelium displaying proliferative tendencies with the spectrum ranging from atypia to dysplasia to carcinoma-in-situ to invasive carcinoma (Fig. 7.1e); however, invasive carcinoma in IPMN, unlike SCN or MCN, is present at the time of diagnosis in 40–50%, thus characterizing this neoplasm as having a more aggressive tumor biology. IPMN has two forms: (1) main duct disease (~80%) that involves the main pancreatic duct with or without secondary changes in the side branches about a third of the time; and (2) side-branch disease (~20%) with involvement only of a segmental branch(es) of the main duct. Invasive carcinoma is present less commonly (only 10–15%) in the side-branch variant.

# Differentiation of Cystic Pancreatic Lesions

Several concepts are crucial in diagnosing patients with cystic lesions of the pancreas – differentiation of non-neoplastic from neoplastic, differentiation of serous from mucinous neoplasms, and differentiation of MCN from IPMN.

## Clinical Presentation

Pseudocysts always arise in patients with previous pancre-atopathy – acute or chronic pancreatitis. Although cystic neoplasms can cause pancreatitis, especially IPMN, the lack of previous pancreatic symptoms strongly suggests neoplasm, and a cystic lesion in the pancreas without a previous history of pancreatic pathology should be considered to be a cystic neoplasm until proven otherwise.

## Imaging

The most common imaging modalities currently are US and CT, both of which can help to differentiate the spectrum of cystic pancreatic lesions, but MRCP is also useful if available. Transabdominal US is often the first test suggestive of the diagnosis, but usually a CT is also needed to image adequately the rest of the abdomen, stage the disease, and better visual-ize the pancreas. Cystic neoplasms usually lack inflammatory changes surrounding the lesion, and the pancreatic paren-chyma of the non-involved gland looks normal. SCNs (Fig. 7.2a) appear as a honeycomb of small cysts, often with a central, starburst-like calcified scar (30%). On occasion, the mass may appear "solid" on CT due to the microscopic cysts, but the "cystic" component should be evident on US and especially on endoscopic ultrasonography (EUS). Oligocystic SCNs (one large cyst) exist, but are very rare. In general, SCNs have > 6 cysts/neoplasm with individual cysts < 2 cm in diameter. Endoscopic retrograde cholangio-pancreatography (ERCP) is usually not indicated, and no communication with cystic mass will be shown.

In contrast, MCNs (Fig. 7.2b, c) appear as a well-defined, rounded cystic mass composed of multiple cysts (usually < 6 per neoplasm) each of >2 cm. Ostensibly, a single cyst maybe evident, but often this cyst will have a septum or papillary infolding. The vast majority of MCNs do not communicate with the pancreatic duct, and thus, ERCP is of little value.

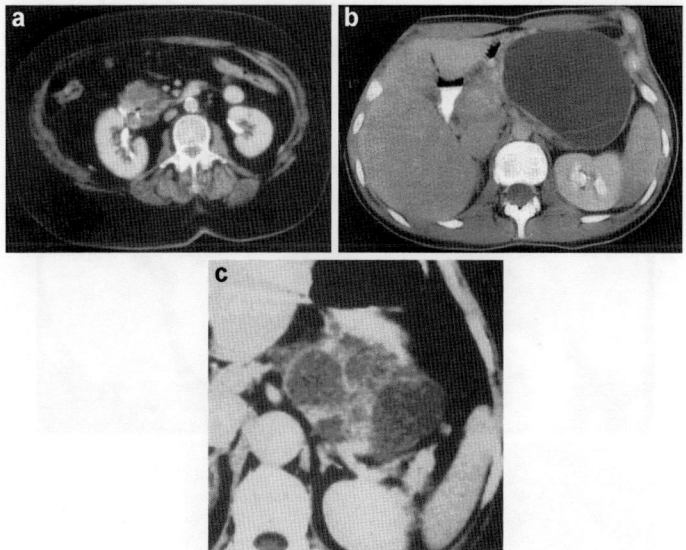

FIGURE 7.2. CTs of primarily cystic neoplasms. (**a**) SCN – note central calcification and multiple small cysts. (**b, c**) MCN – note apparent single cyst (**b**), but with a spectrum of larger cysts in (**c**) (**a** and **b** reprinted from Sarretal., 2003. Reproduced with permission from the Society for Surgery of the Alimentary Tract).

Important considerations are signs of invasive cancer, which include focal extracystic changes or an eccentric-based mass in or around the cystic lesion.

Imaging of *IPMN* is more diverse and demanding. On US, findings include a dilated pancreatic duct and/or an apparent multicystic lesion(s). CT most characteristically shows a dilated main pancreatic duct, either segmentally dilated in the proximal or distal gland or dilated throughout the gland (Fig. 7.3). In branch-duct disease, the main pancreatic duct is normal, but a focal, multi-cystic lesion resembling a bunch of grapes, can be seen, most commonly occurring in the head or uncinate process of the gland and rarely in multiple areas throughout the gland. Side-branch disease may be misinterpreted as MCN, yet MCNs are more rounded, while

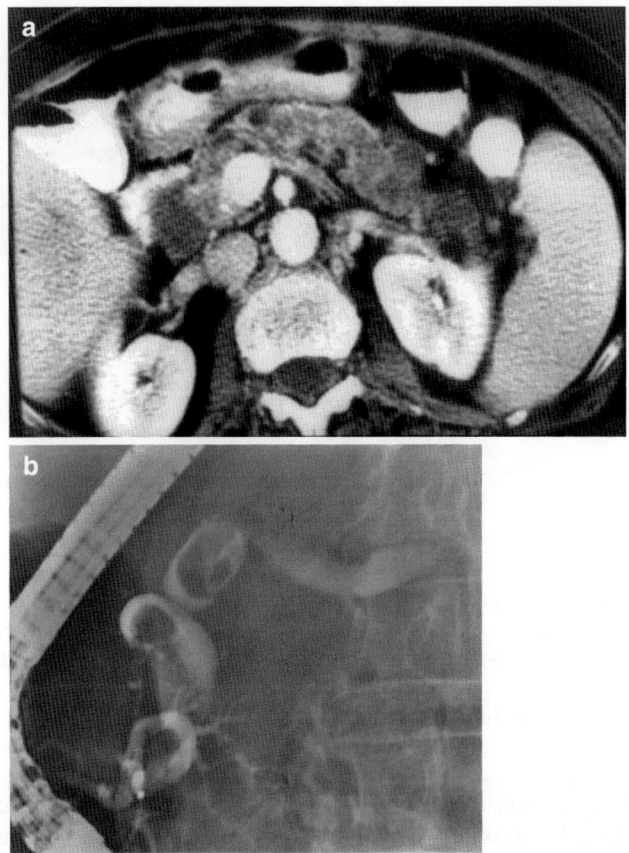

FIGURE 7.3. IPMN. (a) CT shows a markedly dilated main pancreatic duct, confirmed on ERCP (b) (Reprinted from Loftus et al.,
1996. Copyright 1996. With permission from the American
Gastroenterological Association).

branch-duct IPMN is more lobulated. ERCP (and MRCP) in
IPMN shows direct communication with the pancreatic ductal system; in addition, visual inspection of the ampulla may
show mucous exuding from the papilla. IPMN with an invasive carcinoma may have certain features. The presence of a
solid-based mass within the cystic lesion or extrahepatic

biliary obstruction related to the cystic lesion should alert the surgeon to this possibility. EUS is of considerable help, because the presence of mural nodules > 3mm suggests malignancy. Positron emission tomography (PET) appears to be promising but is expensive and requires more work to determine its real usefulness.

## Cyst-Fluid Evaluation

Analysis of percutaneous or endoscopically aspirated fluid may be of benefit. A high amylase activity in the fluid may differentiate inflammatory pseudocysts from SCN and MCN, but the clinician must be wary, because IPMN arises from the pancreatic duct and will have an increased fluid amylase. Cytologic evaluation is helpful if mucinous cells, mucin, an increased viscosity, or the concentration of CEA (carcinoembryonic antigen) is increased (~>250 ng/ml), because these findings differentiate mucinous (potentially malignant) from serous (benign) lesions. However, if the fluid does not reveal these findings, the results are less reliable. Note that cytologic exam for malignant cells is helpful only if positive but is not at all reliable if negative.

## Treatment

Treatment varies with the type of cystic neoplasm, and thus preoperative differentiation and correct preoperative diagnosis is very important.

## SCN

Because these neoplasms are benign, operative resection may not be necessary, especially in the asymptomatic or elderly patient, and especially if resection will require pancreatoduodenectomy. Such an expectant, non-operative approach does have some limitations: (1) the diagnosis of SCN may be inaccurate, overlooking a mucinous neoplasm (MCN, IPMN); (2) SCNs can grow and cause future symptoms – recent evidence suggests that SCNs greater than 4 cm are at higher risk of more rapid growth and may warrant a more aggressive approach; and (3) patients must understand the risks. Symptomatic SCN is an indication for an anatomic, localized resection; enucleation appears to have a higher rate of complications. None recur after complete resection.

## MCN

Because MCNs are all at least "potentially" malignant, ideally all MCNs should be resected. Large series show that about 40% have severe-enough changes of dysplasia and carcinoma-in-situ (often called proliferative or borderline) that they are "premalignant" and warrant an aggressive approach. True cystadeno*carcinomas* with tissue invasion are less common, and despite curative resection, still behave aggressively with 5-year survivals of <50%.When completely resected with tumor-free margins and no areas of tissue invasion (despite changes of dysplasia and carcinoma-in-situ), recurrence approaches zero and follow up surveillance imaging is not necessary. Resections should involve formal anatomic resections; attempts at enucleation or some of the non-anatomic, duodenum-preserving, subtotal head resections are not suggested, because some investigators have shown markers of potential malignancy in the immediately adjacent normal, uninvolved pancreatic parenchyma, raising the question of a generalized field defect.

## IPMN

Although most surgeons would consider IPMN itself to be an indication for resection, the ideal type of surgical resection remains somewhat debatable. Some evidence suggests that

IPMN may involve a global abnormality of *all* pancreatic ductal epithelium, thus questioning by some groups the need for total pancreatectomy to prevent recurrence. For main duct disease, most pancreatic surgeons, however, treat IPMN with a site-directed, formal anatomic resection (proximal, central, or distal pancreatectomy based on location of disease) and a "creeping" further resection should the margin prove to be involved by IPMN. Total pancreatectomy, with its postoperative sequelae of the apancreatic state, is thus reserved for IPMN involving the entire main duct (~20%). For side-branch disease, again a site-directed, anatomic resection is indicated. Because of the 15–50% risk of invasive carcinoma and the origin from the ductal system, enucleation or non-anatomic resections are not appropriate. As for pancreatic ductal carcinoma, extended lymphadenectomy is of unproven benefit.

However, unlike for SCN or MCN, postoperative surveillance for recurrence after resection of IPMN is necessary. The best modalities for postoperative imaging include CT and especially EUS. Even after resection of IPMN without any tissue invasion and a tumor-free ductal margin, recurrence in the remnant pancreas may occur in up to 5–10% of patients. After resection for IPMN with an invasive focus of cancer, however, recurrence approaches 50–60%; thus, although curative survival after curative resection of IPMN is better than after typical ductal cancer of the pancreas, IPMN with invasion is still an aggressive disease. Adjuvant chemo-radiation therapy, while usually suggested, is of unproven benefit.

# Selected Readings

Chari ST, Yadav D, Smyrk TC, DiMagno EP, Miller LJ, Raimondo M, Clain JE, Norton IA, Pearson RK, Petersen BT, Wiersema MJ, Farnell MB, Sarr MG (2002) Study of recurrence after surgical resection of intraductal papillary mucinous neoplasm of the pancreas. Gastroenterology 123:1500–1507

Loftus EV Jr, Olivares-Pakzad BA, Batts KP, et al. (1996) Intraductal papillary-mucinous tumors of the pancreas: clinicopathologic features, outcome, and nomenclature. Gastroenterology 110:1909–1918

Pyke CM, van Heerden JA, Colby TV, Sarr MG, Weaver AL (1992) The spectrum of serous cystadenoma of the pancreas: clinical, pathological, and surgical aspects. Ann Surg 215:132–139

Salvia R, Fernandez-del Castillo C, Bassi C, Thayer SP, Falconi M, Mantovani W, Pederzoli P, Warshaw AL (2004) Main-duct intraductal papillary mucinous neoplasms of the pancreas: clinical predictors of malignancy and long-term survival following resection. Ann Surg 239:678–687

Sarr MG, Carpenter HA, Prabhakar LP, Orchard TF, Hughes S, van Heerden JA, DiMagno EP (2000) Clinical and pathologic correlation of 84 mucinous cystic neoplasms of the pancreas – can one reliably differentiate benign from malignant (or premalignant) neoplasms? Ann Surg 231:205–212

Sarr MG, Murr M, Smyrk TC, Yeo CJ, Fernandez-del Castillo C, Hawes RH, Freeny PC (2003) Primary cystic neoplasms of the pancreas: neoplastic disorders of emerging importance – current state-of-the-art and unanswered questions. J Gastrointest Surg 7:417–428

# Part II
# Pancreas — Malignant

# 8
# Pancreatic Carcinoma

**Melinda M. Mortenson, Debra L. Kennamer, Eric P. Tamm, Huamin Wang, and Douglas B. Evans**

## Pearls and Pitfalls

- The majority of patients with a malignant-appearing stricture of the intrapancreatic portion of the bile duct and a low density mass on computed tomography (CT) images will have a malignant pancreatic or periampullary neoplasm.
- Chemotherapy and radiation should not be delivered without tissue confirmation of malignancy.
- Pre-treatment imaging with high quality, contrast-enhanced multidetector CT can stage accurately the extent of disease as resectable (Stages I and II), locally advanced (stage III), or metastatic (stage IV).
- CT criteria for local tumor resectability include absence of tumor extension to the superior mesenteric artery (SMA) and celiac axis, as well as a patent superior mesenteric-portal vein (SMPV) confluence.
- Borderline resectable pancreatic neoplasms are defined as tumors which encase a short segment of the hepatic artery without extension to the celiac axis amenable to resection and reconstruction, tumor abutment of the SMA, or short-segment occlusion of the superior mesenteric vein (SMV), portal vein (PV), or SMPV confluence which is amenable to vascular reconstruction. These patients are at high risk

K.I. Bland et al. (eds.), *Surgery of the Pancreas and Spleen*, DOI: 10.1007/978-1-84996-369-5_8,
© Springer-Verlag London Limited 2011

for positive resection margins and should, in general, receive systemic therapy and chemoradiation prior to resection.

- Perform CT prior to any interventional endoscopic procedure such as endoscopic retrograde cholangiopancreatography (ERCP) or endoscopic ultrasonography (EUS) as post-procedure pancreatitis can distort the pancreatic and periampullary anatomy, prevent the diagnosis of malignant tumor if one exists, and interfere with assessment of the extent of disease.
- Aberrant arterial anatomy should be identified preoperatively on CT and confirmed at the time of surgery. A replaced or accessory right hepatic artery should be identified prior to division of the bile duct.
- Operative exploration should not be used for diagnosis. The operative plan should be clearly delineated prior to going to the operating room based on preoperative imaging.
- The uncinate process should be completely removed from the SMV, and the SMPV confluence mobilized fully to facilitate safe exposure of the SMA. If the SMA is exposed and visualized by the surgeons on both sides of the table it is unlikely to be injured.
- All perineural and soft tissue to the right of the SMA should be removed with the pancreaticoduodenectomy specimen. The inferior pancreaticoduodenal arteries should be identified and ligated individually at their origin from the SMA. Simple ligation of these arteries with a mass of mesenteric tissue may predispose to postoperative hemorrhage.
- A standardized pathologic evaluation of the pancreaticoduodenectomy specimen is necessary. The SMA margin consists of the tissue to the right of the proximal 3–4 cm of the SMA and must be assessed to determine R status.
- Surgeons should be aware of the clinical trials available in their medical center for patients with localized pancreatic cancer (Stages I, II, and III).

# Introduction

Pancreatic cancer is the fourth leading cause of cancer-related death for both men and women in the United States today with an estimated 33,730 people diagnosed with the disease in 2006. For those patients with resectable pancreatic cancer, the long-term survival rate is approximately 20%, and the median survival is approximately 2 years; however, this accounts for only 15–20% of patients diagnosed with the disease. Despite pancreaticoduodenectomy, disease recurs commonly, the most common sites being the liver, lung, peritoneal cavity, and pancreatic tumor bed. Because exocrine pancreatic cancer is characterized by early vascular and lymphatic dissemination, it is likely that subclinical metastases are present in most patients at the time of diagnosis, even when findings from imaging studies suggest localized disease. If the primary tumor is unresectable, the median survival is 9–12 months for patients with locally advanced, inoperable disease and 4–6 months for those with distant metastases.

Patients with pancreatic cancer often present with jaundice at diagnosis secondary to extrahepatic biliary obstruction. Tumors in a location that cause biliary obstruction early in the disease course may be associated with a better prognosis due to earlier diagnosis. In contrast, those patients with tumors that do not cause obstruction are often not diagnosed until they are locally advanced or metastatic. If jaundice is not present, patient complaints are often nonspecific and may include pain, fatigue, weight loss, anorexia, hyperglycemia, and diarrhea due to pancreatic exocrine insufficiency. The pain due to locally infiltrative pancreatic cancer is typically a dull, constant, poorly localized visceral pain in the middle and upper back secondary to invasion of the celiac and mesenteric plexus.

The extent of disease is best categorized as resectable (Stage I or II), locally advanced (Stage III), or metastatic (Stage IV). The TNM staging system has been modified in the last edition of the AJCC Cancer Staging Manual due to the availability of pretreatment imaging that allows staging to be based on high quality CT images and reflects the importance of stage-specific treatment planning.

In this chapter, we review our current approach to the diagnosis and surgical treatment of patients with localized pancreatic cancer. Good surgical outcomes require proper patient selection, detailed surgical technique, and attention to all aspects of patient care especially anesthetic management. Due to space limitations, we will not be able to comment on the expanding field of adjuvant and neoadjuvant therapy and refer the reader to a recent review by our group.

## Epidemiology

The risk factors for pancreatic cancer are a complex interaction between genetic and environmental factors. Age is clearly a factor with the risk of pancreatic cancer increasing sharply after the age of 50. While pancreatic cancer was more common in men than women in the past, currently the incidence is about the same for both sexes in the United States. Trends in incidence and mortality are similar worldwide, although there are slight regional and ethnic differences. Incidence rates are highest in industrialized societies and western countries. In the United States, rates are particularly high in native Hawaiians, Korean Americans, and African Americans, while in Europe rates are highest in Nordic countries.

Genetic syndromes associated with an increased risk of pancreatic cancer include hereditary pancreatitis (often due to mutations in the trypsinogen gene, PRSS1) and the Peutz-Jeghers syndrome (due to a mutation in the STK11/LKB1 gene coding for a serine threonine kinase). Other than these very rare conditions, high-risk groups can not really be found. The incidence of pancreatic cancer is low in the general population (0.01%), however, recently identified patient subsets with a modest increase in risk include BRCA2 mutation carriers (tenfold), those with mutations in p16 (20-fold), and those thought to have a strong family history of pancreatic cancer (13-fold). The increase in risk is fairly minimal and the conditions rare, therefore, a sizable population of high-risk patients suitable for careful analysis does not exist. It is controversial whether there is a causal association between the development of pancreatic cancer and diabetes mellitus or chronic pancreatitis.

Smoking clearly increases the risk of pancreatic cancer. The risk increases with greater tobacco use up to a relative risk ratio of 10 in those smoking greater than two packs per day. Variations in the gender and ethnic incidence of pancreatic cancer may be due to changes in tobacco use in these groups. Dietary factors also contribute to increased risk. The risk increases in those with diets high in animal protein and fat, salt, smoked or barbequed meats, and refined foods and sugars; the risk decreases with consumption of fruit and vegetables.

## Molecular Biology

A multitude of interacting signaling pathways are involved in the transformation of a pancreatic duct cell into cancer. A model of the histologic and genetic progression of pancreatic ductal adenocarcinoma has been developed analogous to that shown for colorectal carcinoma but of much greater complexity. Precursor lesions arise in the pancreatic ducts beginning with the histologic appearance of pancreatic intraepithelial neoplasia (PanIN). Activating mutations in *K-ras* and *Her-2/neu* occur early, loss of p16 expression occurs in intermediate lesions, and inactivation of *p53*, *BRCA2*, and *DPC4* occur later in the malignant transformation of duct cells.

Targeted therapy directed toward the aberrant molecular pathways in pancreatic cancer offers hope for improved response rates. Multiple targeted therapeutic agents have been developed, including inhibitors of metalloproteinases, farnesyl transferases, the NF-κB pathway, tyrosine kinases, and growth factor receptors. Vascular endothelial growth factor (VEGF) is a proangiogenic molecule overexpressed commonly in pancreatic cancer. This overexpression correlates with more advanced disease. Agents targeting VEGF and downstream signaling pathways are under active development. Epidermal growth factor receptor (EGFR) is detected in greater than 90% of pancreatic cancers and elevated expression levels of EGFR predict poor prognosis. A multi-center phase III trial combining cetuximab, a chimeric antibody against EGFR, and gemcitabine is in progress. Erlotinib, a small molecule tyrosine kinase inhibitor, combined with gemcitabine has been shown to improve survival in patients with metastatic pancreatic cancer compared to gemcitabine alone. The treatment is generally well-tolerated with rash being the most common side effect (72%).

## Diagnostic Evaluation

Preoperative evaluation of the patient with suspected or biopsy-proven pancreatic cancer includes physical examination, routine laboratory testing, chest radiography, and contrast-enhanced, multi-detector CT of the abdomen and pelvis. We advocate careful pretreatment staging based on objective CT criteria to define potentially resectable pancreatic cancer (Fig. 8.1). These criteria include: (1) absence of tumor extension to the SMA, celiac axis, and common hepatic artery (CHA); (2) patent SMPV confluence; and (3) absence of metastatic disease. Locally advanced, unresectable neoplasms are defined as those that encase the celiac axis and/or SMA (Fig. 8.2) or that occlude the SMV, PV, or SMPV confluence (Table 8.1). The term "encasement" describes a vessel-tumor relationship in which a tumor is inseparable from the vessel for >180° of the circumference of the vessel. If the tumor is inseparable from the vessel for ≤180° of the circumference of the vessel, we use the term "abutment."

The term "borderline resectable" has been developed for those neoplasms in which it is difficult to distinguish between resectable and locally advanced disease. Such neoplasms, if resected, usually involve a more complex pancreatic resection often including vascular resection and reconstruction. Criteria we use to define borderline resectable pancreatic

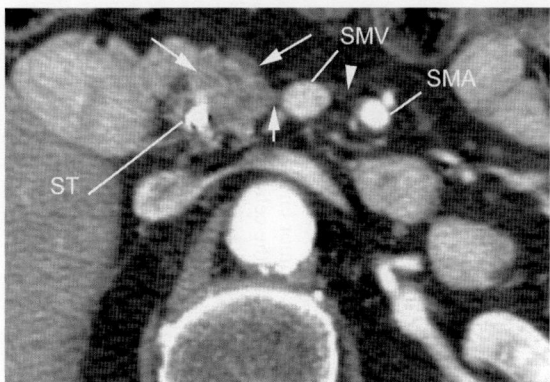

FIGURE 8.1. Axial contrast-enhanced CT image from the pancreatic parenchymal phase of a resectable pancreatic cancer (long white arrows) that contacts (short white arrow) the superior mesenteric vein (SMV) but is separated from the superior mesenteric artery (SMA) by an intact tissue plane (white arrowhead). Resection and reconstruction of a portion of the superior mesenteric vein may be necessary. A biliary stent is also present (ST).

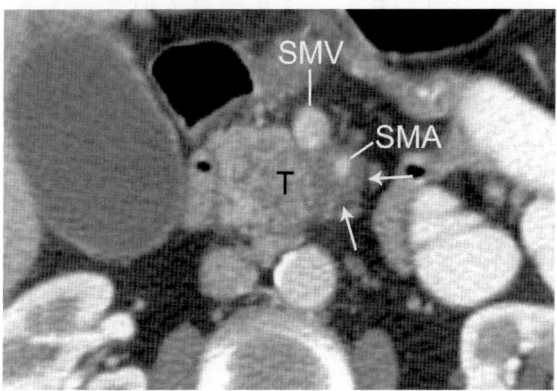

FIGURE 8.2. Axial contrast-enhanced CT image of a locally advanced pancreatic cancer (black T) due to encasement of the superior mesenteric artery (SMA). The medial extent of the tumor is identified by the arrows. The superior mesenteric vein (SMV) is anterior and lateral to the SMA.

TABLE 8.1. MD Anderson definitions for the preoperative staging of localized pancreatic cancer.

| Vessel | Resectable | Borderline resectable | Locally advanced |
|---|---|---|---|
| SMA | Normal tissue plane between tumor and vessel | Tumor abutment ≤ 180 or ≤ 50% of the circumference of the artery | Tumor encasement (>180°) |
| Celiac axis/common hepatic artery | Normal tissue plane between tumor and vessel | Short-segment encasement or abutment of the common hepatic artery (typically at the gastroduodenal origin) | Tumor encasement (>180°) of the celiac axis |
| SMV/PV | Patent SMV/PV confluence | Short-segment occlusion with suitable vessel above and below to allow for resection and reconstruction | Occlusion with no technical option for reconstruction |

SMA, superior mesenteric artery; SMV/PV, superior mesenteric vein/portal vein.

cancer include: (1) short segment encasement of the hepatic artery without celiac axis involvement that is amenable to resection and reconstruction; (2) abutment of the SMA; or (3) short-segment occlusion of the SMV, PV, or SMPV confluence with a patent SMV below and a patent PV above the area of tumor involvement allowing for vascular reconstruction if necessary. As these patients are at high risk for positive margins, we routinely utilize a multimodality treatment approach involving preoperative (neoadjuvant) chemotherapy usually followed by chemoradiation.

If a low-density mass is not seen on CT, patients with suspected pancreatic cancer should undergo upper endoscopy and EUS which may be able to define a mass not seen on CT. Because procedure-induced pancreatitis may interfere with accurate assessment of disease on CT, interventional endoscopy should only be performed after the CT is completed. If the EUS does not demonstrate a tumor and the patient has biliary obstruction, ERCP is performed. At the time of ERCP, a malignant obstruction of the intrapancreatic portion of the bile duct can often be accurately differentiated from a benign bile duct stricture. During diagnostic ERCP in patients with extrahepatic biliary obstruction, endobiliary stents are placed routinely to prevent cholangitis. In addition, stents are placed in patients with increased bilirubin levels in whom operation is expected to be delayed, including those enrolled in clinical trials involving preoperative chemotherapy or chemoradiation. Furthermore, if the duration of preoperative therapy is expected to be greater than 6–8 weeks, an expandable metal stent should be considered to prevent endobiliary stent occlusion and the need for stent exchange while the patient is receiving chemotherapy.

Currently, the procedure of choice for obtaining a cytologic diagnosis of a malignant neoplasm in patients with non-metastatic pancreatic neoplasms and an identifiable pancreatic mass is EUS-guided fine needle aspiration (FNA). Confirmation of malignancy is required in all patients with locally advanced or metastatic disease prior to treatment with systemic therapy or radiation and is necessary in patients with resectable disease who are to receive protocol-based preoperative chemotherapy or chemoradiation. False-negative results may occur, especially when biopsy is attempted on small tumors, and therefore negative results from EUS-guided FNA should not be considered definite proof that a malignancy does not exist.

Many surgeons will perform laparoscopy routinely at the same anesthesia induction as a planned laparotomy when considering major pancreatic resection for presumed localized, resectable pancreatic cancer. Diagnostic laparoscopy is easily performed and detects the 10–15% of patients that may have occult extrapancreatic metastatic disease not recognized on CT, thereby preventing these patients from undergoing a nontherapeutic laparotomy. In contrast, local tumor resectability should be determined at the time of preoperative CT imaging and laparotomy should not be used just to assess the possibility of local tumor resection. It is no longer acceptable to perform a major laparotomy in patients with presumed pancreatic cancer just to "explore" the possibility of resection.

# Anesthetic Management for Major Pancreatic Resection

Unless contraindicated, a mid to low thoracic epidural catheter is placed prior to induction of general anesthesia and is activated with either a local anesthetic alone or combined with an opiate prior to the surgical incision. This is followed by a continuous infusion of low concentration local anesthetic throughout the procedure. General inhalational anesthesia is maintained in combination with an opiate infusion and muscle relaxant. The patients volume status is closely monitored with continuous arterial and venous pressure monitors and a urine output of 1–2 ml/kg/h is acceptable. Forced warm air is used to maintain the patients body temperature at 37°C. Unless the patient has a severe pre-existing cardiopulmonary co-morbidity, the patient is extubated and remains in a monitored setting overnight prior to transfer to the surgical ward. Patient controlled epidural anesthesia (PCEA) is then maintained for 3–4 days postoperatively.

Patient satisfaction scores are higher in patients receiving PCEA compared to intravenous patient-controlled analgesia (PCA) with improved pain relief both at rest and with coughing. In addition, PCEA is associated with shorter times to extubation, improved pulmonary dynamics, and more rapid return of bowel activity. Data also suggest a physiologic and clinical benefit to PCEA beyond that of just improved pain control. The combination of epidural and general anesthesia followed by PCEA increases wound tissue oxygenation, an important determinant of wound healing, likely due to the vasodilatory properties of the local anesthetics as well as the decreased physiologic stress response to surgery. The stress due to surgery and postoperative pain likely contribute to perioperative immunosuppression due to complex interactions between the nervous and immune systems. Patients receiving a mixture of opiates and local anesthetics via PCEA may have less immunosuppression, the clinical significance of which remains an active area of investigation.

## Pancreaticoduodenectomy

Our recommended technique for pancreaticoduodenectomy usually begins with a diagnostic laparoscopy followed by a midline, or occasionally, a bilateral subcostal incision depending on patient anatomy. The abdomen is explored carefully first with the laparoscope and then after opening the abdomen to exclude extrapancreatic metastatic disease. In general, we do not perform random lymph node sampling for frozen section analysis intraoperatively. Each patient should be considered individually, however; for example, in a high-risk patient (advanced age, significant medical co-morbidities, high serum level of CA19-9, etc.) with suspicious adenopathy, a positive regional lymph node may be viewed as a contraindication to proceeding with pancreaticoduodenectomy.

We favor the pylorus-preserving technique in patients at risk for nutritional depletion, which can occur after standard pancreaticoduodenectomy (to include distal gastrectomy and gastrojejunostomy) due to increased gastrointestinal transit potentiated by rapid gastric emptying out of the gastroje-junostomy. Pylorus preservation may allow for more controlled gastric emptying, reduced transit time, and enhanced intestinal absorption. Thin patients, especially if of advanced age, may benefit most from preservation of the pylorus and we attempt to preserve the pylorus in such patients with small periampullary or duodenal tumors. Pylorus preservation should not be performed in patients with bulky pancreatic head neoplasms, duodenal neoplasms involving the first portion of the duodenum, or lesions associated with grossly positive pyloric or peripyloric lymph nodes.

The surgical resection can be divided into six defined steps facilitating organization of such a complex operation, minimizing operative time, and providing a clear operative plan to trainees who may still be in the early phases of the learning curve.

## Step one: Exposure of the SMV

The lesser sac is entered and the hepatic flexure of the colon is reflected inferiorly thereby separating the colon (and its mesentery) from the duodenum and pancreatic head. One can then expose the anterior surface of the infrapancreatic SMV at the level of the pancreatic neck. The mesentery along the inferior border of the pancreas from a point medial to the middle colic vessels is incised and carried out laterally and inferiorly to expose the junction of the middle colic vein and the SMV. The middle colic vein may enter directly into the anterior surface of the infrapancreatic SMV or arise as a common trunk with the gastroepiploic vein (gastrocolic trunk). If the middle colic vein and gastroepiploic vein share a common trunk, the common trunk is divided; otherwise, the gastroepiploic vein is left intact and divided later in the operation after pancreatic transection. When necessary, the middle colic vein can also be divided.

## Step two: Kocher maneuver

In contrast to how many mobilize the duodenum and pancreatic head, we begin the dissection at the transverse portion (third portion) of the duodenum by identifying the inferior vena cava (IVC); one can therefore refer to this as a "reverse Kocher". We prefer to begin low at the level of the transverse portion of the duodenum as it allows for early identification of the IVC and is a more anatomic procedure. All fibrofatty and lymphatic tissue antero-medial to the right gonadal vein and anterior to the IVC is elevated, along with the pancreatic head and duodenum. The right gonadal vein serves as a good landmark to help prevent inadvertent injury to the ureter which is usually lateral and slightly posterior to the gonadal vein. Dissection is continued to the left lateral edge of the aorta, with care to identify the left renal vein. An accessory right renal artery (which is an end artery) may occasionally course anterior to the IVC on its way to the right kidney; this vessel should be preserved. Manual palpation of the tumor at this time is not necessary; palpation is an inaccurate way to assess the relationship of the tumor to the SMA. The relationship of the pancreatic tumor to the SMA is the major focus of the preoperative imaging evaluation.

## Step three: Portal dissection

The portal dissection begins by exposure of the common hepatic artery (CHA). The CHA is exposed by removing the large lymph node which lies directly anterior to this vessel. The right gastric artery and then the gastroduodenal artery (GDA) are ligated and divided. Even if we are planning pylorus-preservation, we still prefer to ligate the right gastric artery to allow for greater mobilization of the distal stomach and pyloric region. If tumor extension to within a few millimeters of the GDA is present, one should obtain proximal and distal control of the hepatic artery and divide the GDA flush at its origin. Careful sharp dissection and vascular control will prevent intimal dissection of the hepatic artery. The common/proper hepatic artery is then mobilized off of the underlying PV which can be found within the triangle formed by the CHA, GDA, and superior border of the pancreas. The gallbladder is removed from the gallbladder fossa and the common hepatic duct is transected at its junction with the cystic duct. Before dividing the common hepatic duct, we recommend doing three things: first, insure that the portal vein is well exposed, second, re-establish the foramen of Winslow (if it was obliterated due to adhesions) to allow palpation of the porta hepatis, and finally, with the left index finger in the foramen of Winslow, confirm the presence or absence of an aberrant hepatic artery posterior to the bile duct and posterolateral to the portal vein. The bile (hepatic) duct is then divided and when possible, a gentle bulldog clamp is placed on the transected bile duct to prevent bile spillage.

## Step four: Division of the stomach or duodenum

Transection of the stomach is performed with a linear gastrointestinal stapler so as to perform a standard antrectomy. When opening the lesser omentum, be aware that an accessory left hepatic artery may be present arising from the left gastric artery. Overly aggressive division of the lesser omentum in a proximal direction may injure this vessel. If a pylorus-preserving pancreaticoduodenectomy is to be performed, the duodenum is divided 2–3 cm from the pylorus and the gastroepiploic arcade divided at that level. As mentioned above, we divide the right gastric artery even when performing a pylorus-preserving pancreaticoduodenectomy which makes preservation of the gastroepiploic artery (based on the short gastric vessels), and left gastric artery very important.

## Step five: Division of the mesentery of the proximal jejunum and distal duodenum

The loose attachments of the ligament of Treitz are taken down with care to avoid injury to the inferior mesenteric vein. The jejunum is transected approximately 10 cm distal to the ligament of Treitz. We prefer to tie the mesenteric side (staying side) of the proximal jejunum and duodenum and use the harmonic scalpel on the serosal (bowel) side. The devascularized jejunum and duodenum are then reflected beneath the mesenteric vessels.

## Step six: Division of the pancreas and separation of the specimen from the SMPV confluence and the SMA

The pancreas is transected using electrocautery at the level of the SMPV confluence. Proper mobilization of the SMV involves identification of the jejunal branch of the SMV which originates from the right posterolateral aspect of the SMV at the level of the uncinate process, travels posterior to the SMA, and enters the medial (proximal) aspect of the jejunal mesentery (Fig. 8.3). The few venous tributaries to the uncinate process, arising from the jejunal branch of the SMV are divided. The uncinate process should be removed completely from the SMV. This allows safe exposure of the SMA by medial retraction of the SMPV confluence. The specimen is then separated from the right lateral wall of the SMA, which is dissected to its origin at the aorta (Fig. 8.4). Exposure of the SMA is necessary for direct ligation of the inferior pancreaticoduodenal arteries (usually two of them). Mass ligation of these vessels with mesenteric soft tissue is the major cause of postoperative retroperitoneal hemorrhage, because this vessel may retract from a poorly placed tie or ligature. In addition, direct exposure of the SMA allows for removal of all mesenteric soft tissue and perineural tissue to the right of this vessel. The high incidence of local recurrence after pancreaticoduodenectomy mandates that greater attention be paid to the SMA margin (the soft tissue margin along the right lateral border of the proximal 3–4 cm of the SMA).

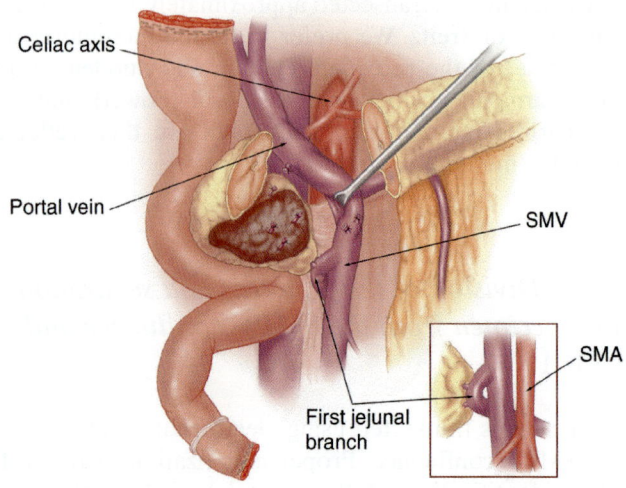

FIGURE 8.3. Illustration of the important surgical anatomy of the superior mesenteric vein (SMV) at the level of the uncinate process. The SMV usually bifurcates into two main branches, one to the ileum and one to the jejunum. Adequate venous return from the small bowel requires that one or the other of these two main SMV-tributaries is intact. The jejunal branch of the SMV (often referred to as the first jejunal branch) drains the proximal jejunum, travels posterior to the superior mesenteric artery (SMA), and enters the SMV along its posterolateral wall. The jejunal branch usually has a few venous tributaries that drain the uncinate process (inset). If necessary, the jejunal branch can be divided. Very rarely the jejunal branch will travel anterior to the SMA.

## Pathologic Assessment of the Pancreaticoduodenectomy Specimen

The template for the pathology reporting of pancreaticoduo-denectomy specimens currently used at our institution appears in Table 8.2. Such templates are necessary to allow accurate transfer of pathologic data to prospective databases and to ensure a more accurate prognosis. The pathologic evaluation of the pancreaticoduodenectomy specimen begins

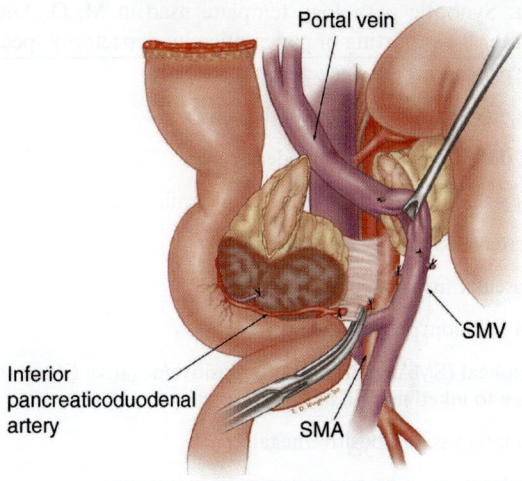

FIGURE 8.4. Illustration of the final step in resection of the specimen. Medial retraction of the superior mesenteric-portal vein confluence facilitates dissection of the soft tissues adjacent to the lateral wall of the proximal superior mesenteric artery (SMA); this site represents the SMA margin. The inferior pancreaticoduodenal artery (or arteries) is identified at its origin from the SMA, ligated, and divided. SMV, superior mesenteric vein.

with frozen-section analysis of the pancreatic and common hepatic/bile duct transection margins, both of which are submitted en-face. Positive resection margins on the hepatic/bile duct or pancreas should be resected to a negative margin if possible. Complete permanent-section analysis of the pancreaticoduodenectomy specimen requires that it be oriented with the pathologist to identify and assess accurately the SMA margin of excision and other standard pathologic variables (Fig. 8.5). The perineural and mesenteric tissue along the proximal SMA represents the SMA margin. Because we remove all tissue to the right of the SMA, further resection at the SMA margin is not possible. The SMA margin of excision is then serially sectioned perpendicular to the inked margin and submitted entirely for histologic examination after overnight fixation.

TABLE 8.2. Synoptic pathology template used at M. D. Anderson cancer center for reporting of pancreaticoduodenectomy specimens.

Specimen: pancreaticoduodenectomy

Tumor diagnosis: histologic type of the tumor

Degree of differentiation: well/moderate/poor

The tumor size: the maximal dimension in centimeters

Extrapancreatic extension: present/absent

Lymphovascular invasion: present/absent

Perineural invasion: present/absent

Retroperitoneal (SMA) margin status: positive/negative (if negative, the distance to inked margin in mm)

Bile duct margin status: positive/negative

Pancreatic transection margin status: positive/negative

Proximal stomach or duodenum margin status: positive/negative

Distal duodenum or jejunum margin status: positive/negative

Regional Lymph Nodes:

   Total number of positive lymph nodes

   Total number of lymph nodes examined

If vessel resection performed:

   Name of the vessel removed

Presence or absence of vessel invasion and the layer of vessel wall involved:

   Perivascular connective tissue/vessel wall/into the lumen

   Vascular resection margin status

Degree of treatment effect (if patient received preoperative therapy): reported as a percentage of viable tumor cells

classified as <10%, 10–50%, 50–90%, >90%[a]

Final pTNM Staging (AJCC 6th edition):

   pT: T1/T2/T3

   pN: N0/N1

   pMX: Distant metastasis

[a]Data from Evans et al. (1992).

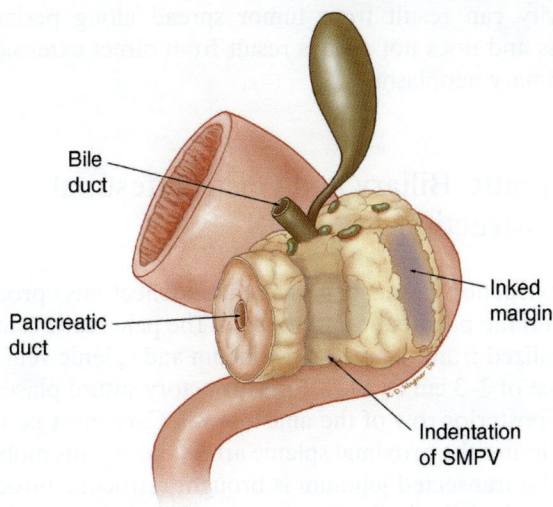

Bile
duct

Inked
margin

Pancreatic
duct

Indentation
of SMPV

FIGURE 8.5. Illustration of a pancreaticoduodenectomy specimen demonstrating how the superior mesenteric artery margin should be inked at the time of permanent section pathologic examination. This margin cannot be retrospectively evaluated if the margin was not inked for identification at the time of gross inspection. SMPV = superior mesenteric-portal vein.

The pathologist cannot usually differentiate an R1 (microscopically positive) from an R2 (grossly positive) SMA margin in the absence of information regarding the retroperitoneal dissection, which should be included in the surgeons operative dictation. The R designation should be listed in the dictated operative report by having the surgeon wait to sign-off on the operative report until the pathology report is available for review and therefore the status of the SMA margin determined. For example, if the surgeon states that gross tumor was encountered when completing the SMA dissection, a positive histologic margin should result in the R2 designation in the operative report and the medical record. If the surgeon states that there was no gross evidence of tumor extension to the SMA margin, then a positive histologic margin should result in the R1 designation. A microscopically positive margin may occur in at least 10–20% of resections; margin positivity can result from tumor spread along perineural sheaths and does not always result from direct extension of the primary neoplasm.

# Pancreatic, Biliary and Gastrointestinal Reconstruction

Reconstruction after pancreaticoduodenectomy proceeds first with the pancreatic anastomosis. The pancreatic remnant is mobilized from the retroperitoneum and splenic vein for a distance of 2–3 cm to allow for satisfactory suture placement of the posterior row of the anastomosis. Care must be taken not to injure the proximal splenic artery during this mobilization. The transected jejunum is brought retrocolic through a generous incision in the transverse mesocolon to the left of the middle colic vessels. A two-layer, end-to-side, duct-to-mucosa pancreaticojejunostomy is performed using 4-0 or 5-0 monofilament suture. If the pancreatic duct is not dilated, a stent may be used. When the pancreatic parenchyma is soft, we often use pledgets for the anterior row of sutures to prevent them from causing a tear in the pancreatic tissue. Another option that can be utilized in the soft pancreas and non-dilated pancreatic duct is to perform a two-layer anastomosis that invaginates the cut end of the pancreas into the jejunum; however, we rarely use this technique, because even a nondilated pancreatic duct can often be anastomosed using the duct-to-mucosa technique.

A single-layer biliary anastomosis is performed using interrupted 4-0 absorbable monofilament sutures. It is important to align the jejunum with the bile duct to avoid tension on the pancreatic and biliary anastomoses. A stent is used rarely in the construction of the hepaticojejunostomy. The biliary anastomosis is followed by an antecolic, end-to-side gastrojejunostomy constructed in two layers. The distance between the biliary and gastric anastomoses should be at least 50 cm, allowing for a tension-free anastomosis and also to prevent bile reflux cholangitis. We prefer an antecolic gastrojejunostomy to prevent possible outlet obstruction caused by the colonic mesentery. A 10-Fr feeding jejunostomy tube may be placed distal to the gastrojejunostomy. We use jejunostomy tubes in those patients who are at high risk for postoperative complications, have experienced significant weight loss prior to operation, and in all patients who undergo a pylorus preserving pancreaticoduodenectomy (due to the increased risk for delayed gastric emptying). We utilize a gastrostomy tube only rarely for postoperative gastric decompression. We no longer place a drain near the pancreatic anastomosis, although this is still performed by many surgeons. Importantly, we place the mobilized falciform ligament (carefully preserved when the abdomen was opened) anterior to the CHA at the level of the GDA stump and posterior to the afferent jejunal limb so as to cover the GDA stump in an attempt to prevent formation of a pseudoaneurysm at the site of the GDA stump in the event of a pancreatic anastomotic leak.

## Post-Operative Survival and the Role for Adjuvant Therapy

Despite a complete resection, disease recurs in at least 80% of patients. Those with negative margins and negative regional lymph nodes have a greater chance for cure. Therefore, there has been a long-standing interest in delivering chemotherapy with or without radiation therapy after (adjuvant) or before (neoadjuvant) surgery. While the optimal choice of adjuvant chemotherapy or chemoradiation remains controversial, recent studies do suggest a modest survival benefit for those patients who receive adjuvant therapy. However, the delivery of postoperative adjuvant therapy often assumes that all patients who underwent pancreaticoduodenectomy received intended postoperative therapy and that all patients also had all gross tumor removed. Single institution studies have reported that at least 25–30% of patients who undergo a curative resection do not receive postoperative therapy for reasons that are disease related (early tumor progression), treatment related (such as delayed recovery from surgery), or patient related (medical co-morbidities, patient refusal). The number of patients who undergo operative resection but have tumor left behind is often not known due to inadequate preoperative imaging, a lack of surgical quality control, and a failure to report accurately the pathologic margins of resection; thus, incomplete resections are likely more common than we think. That said, efforts continue in the design of cooperative group trials to improve quality control and study contemporary cytotoxic agents (largely gemcitabine based) combined with newer targeted therapies which attack known growth factor pathways.

There are many practical and theoretical advantages to preoperative (neoadjuvant) treatment of patients with localized pancreatic cancer. Most compelling is the ability to provide immediate systemic therapy for a disease that is systemic at diagnosis in virtually all patients. A second more practical advantage is improved patient selection for pancreatic surgery – an operation associated with significant patient morbidity even when performed in experienced hands. This improved patient selection arises because patients with rapidly progressive systemic disease are identified as part of the restaging evaluation performed following neoadjuvant treatment prior to planned surgery. In prospective trials, approximately 25% of patients who begin a treatment program of preoperative treatment do not undergo resection of their primary tumor as a consequence of disease progression or evolution of clinically significant medical co-morbidity. These patients are spared the morbidity and prolonged recovery sometimes associated with pancreaticoduodenectomy. In a series of trials performed at our institution, patients who demonstrated disease progression after preoperative chemoradiation had a median survival of only 7 months. Therefore, many institutions have begun to investigate the role of chemotherapy and/or chemoradiation given preoperatively.

# Issues in the Management of Locally Advanced and Metastatic Disease of Importance for the Surgeon

We reserve laparotomy for those patients with potentially resectable disease. Operation in patients with locally advanced or metastatic pancreatic cancer risks perioperative complications or a prolonged recovery time which is of major concern in patients who have a short expected survival duration. We currently favor the use of metal stents in patients with unresectable neoplasms causing biliary obstruction. For patients with duodenal obstruction, duodenal stents are not as uniformly successful and we generally reserve the use of duodenal stents only for those patients who develop duodenal obstruction late in the course of their disease at a time when further specific anticancer therapy is no longer being considered. For patients who develop duodenal obstruction and are candidates for systemic therapy or chemoradiation, we prefer an operative bypass (combined with jejunostomy tube placement) due to the durability of an operative gastrojejunostomy in resolving mechanical gastric outlet obstruction. Importantly, if endoscopic stent placement in the bile duct or duodenum is unsuccessful in a patient with a good performance status who is planned to receive some form of systemic therapy, we favor proceeding with operative bypass without delay. It is a mistake to continue to pursue nonoperative methods of palliation of biliary or gastric outlet obstruction in a patient awaiting treatment (or under active treatment) in whom an initial endoscopic approach has not met with complete success.

## Summary

Detailed preoperative assessment of resectability and precise attention to surgical technique will maximize the benefit that can be achieved from surgery. At present, the best option for physicians to improve the care of patients with pancreatic cancer is to stage the extent of disease accurately and apply stage-specific therapies which are protocol-based whenever possible. Future progress in the treatment of pancreatic cancer will involve techniques for early diagnosis to allow more patients to undergo potentially curative resection, and the development of more effective systemic therapies which may be combined with surgery and radiation therapy. As our understanding of the molecular pathogenesis of pancreatic cancer improves, we may acquire the ability to develop patient-specific treatment programs based on the known mutations in a patients tumor (from an FNA biopsy for example) and the available therapies which target specific oncogenes, tumor suppressor genes, and signaling pathways. Physicians should assume that the surgical management of patients with pancreatic cancer will become increasingly complex as operative therapy is combined with systemic agents of greater physiologic complexity with toxicity profiles which involve not only end-organ function but also the coagulation cascade, platelet function and critical factors effecting wound healing.

# Selected Readings

American Joint Commission on Cancer (2002) Exocrine pancreas. In: Greene FL, Page DL, Fleming ID, et al. (eds) AJCC Cancer Staging Manual. Springer, New York, pp 157–164

Beilin B, Shavit Y, Trabekin E, et al. (2003) The effects of postoperative pain management on immune response to surgery. Anesth Analg 97:822–827

Crane CH, Varadhachary G, Wolff RA, et al. (2006) The argument for pre-operative chemoradiation for localized, radiographically resectable pancreatic cancer. Best Pract Res Clin Gastroenterol 2:365–82

Evans DB, Lee JE, Tamm EP, Pisters PWT (2007) Pancreatic oduodenectomy (Whipple Operation) and total pancreatectomy for cancer. In: Fischer JF (ed) Mastery of Surgery, 5th edn. Lippincott Williams & Wilkins, Philadelphia, pp 1299–1317

Katz MHG, Hwang RF, Fleming JB, Evans DB (2008) TNM staging of pancreatic adenocarcinoma. Tumor-node-metastasis staging of pancreatic adenocarcinoma. CA Cancer J Clin 58:111–25

Raut CP, Tseng JF, Sun CC, et al. (2007) Impact of Resection Status on Pattern of Failure and Survival after Pancreaticoduodenectomy for Pancreatic Adenocarcinoma. Ann Surg 246:52–60

Tseng JF, Raut CP, Lee JE, et al. (2004) Pancreaticoduodenectomy with vascular resection: margin status and survival duration. J Gastrointest Surg 8:935–950

Varadhachary GR, Tamm EP, Abbruzzese JL, et al. (2006) Borderline resectable pancreatic cancer: definitions, management, and role of preoperative therapy. Ann Surg Oncol 13:1035–46

Von Hoff DD, Evans DB, Hruban RH (2005) Pancreatic Cancer, First Edition. Massachusetts: Jones and Bartlett

Wolff RA, Crane CH, Li D, Abbruzzese JL, et al. (2006) Neoplasms of the exocrine pancreas. In: Kufe DW, Bast RC, Hait WN, Hong WK, et al. (eds) Holland-Frei Cancer Medicine, 6th edn. BC Decker, Ontario, pp 1331–1358

# 9
# Nonfunctioning Pancreatic Endocrine Tumors

**Carmen C. Solórzano and Richard A. Prinz**

## Pearls and Pitfalls

- Nonfunctioning pancreatic endocrine tumors (PET) are uncommon neoplasms.
- Nonfunctioning PETs present with symptoms of local growth or may be increasingly found incidentally on radiographic studies.
- Beware of a patient with the diagnosis of unresectable/metastatic pancreatic cancer surviving longer than expected; a PET may be present.
- Nonfunctioning PETs may be cystic on imaging studies.
- Complete resection of nonfunctioning PETs is associated with prolonged survival but recurrences are common and continued surveillance is warranted.
- When metastases are present, few patients can undergo complete resection of the primary and metastases.
- Selected patients with synchronous low volume unresectable liver metastases who have a symptomatic primary may benefit from its removal.
- Surgical treatment of nonfunctioning PETs in patients with MEN-1 should be individualized and aim to remove all visible tumors while preventing the metabolic complications associated with endocrine and exocrine insufficiency.

Pancreatic endocrine tumors (PET) (also called neuroendocrine or islet cell tumors) are uncommon neoplasms. Clinically

K.I. Bland et al. (eds.), *Surgery of the Pancreas and Spleen*, DOI: 10.1007/978-1-84996-369-5_9, © Springer-Verlag London Limited 2011

detectable PETs are found in five cases per million population. Nonfunctioning PETs can account for up to 53% of all PET. Histologically, these tumors are classified as amine precursor uptake and decarboxylation neoplasms (APUDomas) and share cytochemical features with melanoma, pheochromocytoma, carcinoid tumors, and medullary thyroid carcinoma. PET, like other APUDomas, have the capacity to synthesize and secrete polypeptide products with hormone activity. PETs are considered functional if they are associated with a clinical syndrome due to hormone release, or nonfunctioning if not associated with clinical symptoms. Pancreatic polypeptide (PP) producing tumors (PPomas) are included in the latter category, as the hormone generally causes no specific symptoms. The majority of nonfunctioning PETs are malignant as evidenced by local invasion of contiguous organs, lymph node metastases, and/or distant organ metastases. Many small nonfunctioning PETs are now being found incidentally with modern imaging techniques and there may have a more benign course.

## Etiology

To date, no risk factors for development of nonfunctioning PET have been identified. Functioning and nonfunctioning PETs are associated with multiple endocrine neoplasia type 1 (MEN-1) and von Hippel Lindau (VHL). MEN-1 is an autosomal dominant inherited disorder characterized by the development of hyperparathyroidism, pituitary adenomas, and PETs. The MEN-1 syndrome is caused by mutations in the *MEN1* gene, located on chromosome 11. MEN1 mutations are usually inactivating, and often lead to a truncated protein. Currently no clear genotype-phenotype correlation has been identified for MEN-1 patients with MEN1 mutations. PETs can be identified in 30–80% of patients with MEN-1. Gastrinomas and nonfunctioning PETs or PPomas are the most common PETs in patients with MEN-1. Development of metastatic disease in patients with MEN-1 and PET is uncommon before age 30; however, metastasis from PET is a frequent cause of mortality in this patient population.

Investigators have found loss of heterozygosity (LOH) at the *MEN1* locus in pancreatic tumor specimens of patients with sporadic or MEN-1 related functioning and nonfunctioning PETs. This finding suggests that the *MEN1* gene may play a role in the development of sporadic PETs.

VHL is an autosomal dominant inherited disorder characterized by the development of retinal and central nervous system hemangiomas, renal cell carcinomas, pheochromocytomas, and PETs. PETs develop in 15–20% of patients with VHL. The VHL syndrome is due to mutations in the *VHL* gene, located on chromosome 3 (3p25). No genotype-phenotype association for PETs in VHL has been identified. Interestingly, LOH of chromosome 3p and deletion of chromosome 3 have been found and linked to the development of metastatic disease in patients with sporadic PETs. These data suggest that the *VHL* gene may be involved in the development and progression of PETs.

## Histology and Immunohistochemistry

Because tumor biology, prognosis, and treatment strategies are so different, it is extremely important to differentiate PETs from exocrine pancreatic tumors (adenocarcinoma). The histologic features of PETs are very characteristic, but immunohistochemistry remains very important in confirming the diagnosis. General neuroendocrine immunohistochemical markers that may be useful include synaptophysin, chromogranin A (CgA), and neuron-specific enolase (NSE). Some peptides that cause clinical syndromes can be found with immunohistochemistry in nonfunctioning PETs. Specific pancreatic neuroendocrine immunohistochemical markers that can be commonly identified in nonfunctioning PETs include PP, glucagon, insulin-like peptide, somatostatin, and vasoactive intestinal peptide (VIP). Immunohistochemical staining for these peptides does not directly correlate to serum levels of the hormone or to the severity of any clinical symptoms. PET positive staining for these hormones is not a functioning PET unless it secretes the hormone and causes a clinical syndrome. In equivocal cases, electron microscopy of PETs can be helpful in identifying characteristic ultrastructural electron-dense secretory granules.

The majority of nonfunctioning PETs are malignant. Histology of a nonfunctioning PET is not a reliable predictor of its biologic behavior. Only the presence of adjacent organ invasion, nodal or distant metastases is confirmatory of malignancy. Standard histological features such as size, nuclear pleomorphism, mitotic activity, or presence of vascular invasion, are not reliable in predicting malignancy. Since patients with nonfunctioning PETs as a group are at-risk for the development of metastatic disease, all of these tumors should be considered malignant or potentially malignant.

## Serum Markers

A number of serum markers have been evaluated for their utility in the diagnosis and management of patients with nonfunctioning PET. Nonfunctioning PETs can secrete a number of peptide hormones, proteins, and glycoproteins, including PP, CgA, NSE, and the alpha (a-) or beta (b-) subunits of human chorionic gonadotropin (HCG).

Up to 75% of nonfunctioning PETs are associated with elevated serum levels of PP. Nonfunctioning PETs with or without elevated PP (PPomas) do not differ in presentation or biology. Pancreatic polypeptide has been investigated as a marker for patients with MEN-1, and as a marker for metastatic disease in patients with known PETs. Unfortunately, PP measurements have proven to be of limited value in these patients. PP levels correlate poorly with tumor burden, often do not normalize following surgical resection, have wide intra-patient variability, and may often be falsely elevated. Therefore, treatment decisions should not be based solely on PP levels. PP levels can be elevated in patients with functioning PETs as well as in patients with non-pancreatic carcinoid neuroendocrine tumors and in patients with other pancreatic masses. Elevated plasma levels of PP can occur after a meal in normal individuals, as well as in patients with chronic inflammatory disorders, acute diarrhea, chronic renal failure, diabetes, pancreatitis, alcohol abuse, prior bowel resection, and advanced age. On the other hand, PP levels in combination with other neuroendocrine markers, such as CgA, can be more sensitive in the diagnosis of nonfunctioning PETs.

CgA has been suggested by Nobels and colleagues as the best general neuroendocrine serum marker available for the evaluation and management of patients with neuroendocrine tumors. These investigators evaluated serum levels of CgA, NSE, and the alpha subunit of glycoprotein hormones in a series of 211 patients with a variety of neuroendocrine tumors. The concentrations of CgA, NSE, and alpha subunit of glycoprotein hormones were elevated in 50%, 43%, and 24% of patients with neuroendocrine tumors, respectively. Elevated serum CgA levels were detected in 9 of 13 patients (69%) with nonfunctioning PETs. CgA levels also correlated well with tumor burden. However, the specificity of CgA is not equal to that of the hormonal products of other neuroendocrine tumors (parathyroid hormone in patients with hyperparathyroidism, calcitonin in patients with medullary thyroid cancer). When CgA is elevated prior to treatment it can be used to monitor tumor progression and response to therapy.

## Diagnosis, Imaging and Patient Selection

Nonfunctioning PETs typically present in the fourth or fifth decade of life. Patients with a nonfunctioning PET most commonly present with local symptoms from the primary pancreatic tumor or from liver metastases. Nonfunctioning PETs are usually solitary tumors except in patients with MEN-1 in whom they are usually multiple.

The majority of nonfunctioning PETs are in the pancreatic head. Patient presentation can be similar to patients with pancreatic adenocarcinoma with weight loss, anorexia, abdominal/back pain, and jaundice. Nonfunctioning PETs are often larger than a typical adenocarcinoma. It is exceedingly important to consider the possibility of a PET in patients presenting this way. Common signs and symptoms in patients presenting with a nonfunctioning PET are listed in Table 9.1. Patients with MEN-1 associated or sporadic nonfunctioning PETs may also present with incidentally discovered pancreatic masses identified on abdominal imaging studies performed for unrelated reasons. A recent Italian multicenter retrospective study by Gullo et al. found that 64 of 184 (35%) patients with nonfunctioning PETs had their tumor discovered incidentally while undergoing abdominal ultrasonography as part of a routine check-up. These patients were asymptomatic and less likely to present with synchronous liver and lymph node metastases when compared to symptomatic patients.

On high quality multi-slice contrast enhanced Computed Tomography (CT), a PET usually appears hypervascular or hyperdense (Fig. 9.1a). PETs may contain calcifications (Fig. 9.1b), may be hypodense compared to adjacent pancreatic parenchyma similar to pancreatic adenocarcinomas, and may contain cystic components. Because of the lack of specific

TABLE 9.1. Clinical presentation of nonfunctioning pancreatic endocrine tumors.

| Symptoms/signs |
| --- |
| Abdominal pain |
| Nausea/vomiting |
| Fatigue |
| Abdominal mass |
| Back pain |
| Jaundice |
| Weight loss |
| None |

associated hormonal symptoms, the majority of patients with nonfunctioning PET do not present until they have locally advanced, unresectable or metastatic disease (Fig. 9.1b, c).

We currently use CT criteria to define potentially resectable pancreatic tumors. Determination of resectability of the primary tumor is based upon the relationship of the mass to the superior mesenteric artery (SMA), vein (SMV), and celiac axis. Endoscopic ultrasound (EUS) is also used to help image small tumors (especially in patients with MEN-1), to evaluate the adjacent vasculature and, when necessary, to obtain tissue diagnosis. Magnetic resonance imaging (MRI)

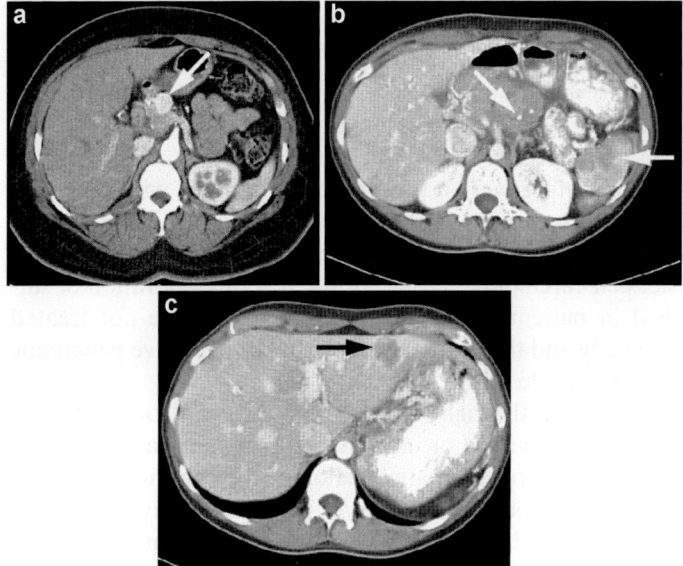

FIGURE 9.1. Abdominal computed tomography (CT) imaging studies of patients with nonfunctioning pancreatic endocrine tumors (PETs). (**a**) An intravenous contrast-enhanced imaging study demonstrating an enhancing mass in the head of the pancreas (arrow). (**b**) A large locally advanced nonfunctioning PET with calcifications involving the celiac axis, SMA and metastatic to a lymph node (white arrows), (**c**) Intravenous contrast-enhanced CT demonstrating a liver metastasis from a PET (black arrow).

with or without pancreatography is used in the presence of a cystic pancreatic neoplasm that needs further characterization, chronic renal insufficiency, or severe contrast allergy. MRI may be more sensitive than CT scan in the detection of liver metastases.

A tumor that encases the celiac axis or the superior mesenteric artery, or causes occlusion of the SMV portal vein confluence without possibility of reconstruction, is considered unresectable. Patients with high volume bilobar liver metastases are also considered unresectable. Some investigators have suggested that "palliative" pancreatic resection (debulking or cytoreductive resection) in patients with unresectable neuroendocrine tumors may provide relief from hormonal or local tumor-related symptoms and improve the efficacy of chemotherapy by decreasing overall tumor burden. However, most of these reports included patients with functioning PETs or carcinoid tumors with syndromes of hormone excess (Table 9.2). There are no available data to support cytoreduction procedures in patients with unresectable nonfunctioning islet cell carcinomas. At this time, we do not advocate incomplete cytoreduction for nonfunctioning islet cell carcinoma because of the favorable duration of survival in patients with locally advanced disease not treated surgically and the potential morbidity of palliative pancreatic resection (vide infra).

Tumors to the right of the SMA and SMV, originating in the pancreatic head or uncinate process, may cause obstruction of the intrapancreatic portion of the common bile duct, gastric outlet obstruction, and/or pain, due to invasion of the retroperitoneal mesenteric plexus. Unlike adenocarcinomas, nonfunctioning PETs occasionally grow to very large size, with minimal symptoms. Patients may have little discomfort and may not develop jaundice, despite the enormous size of these tumors.

PETs rising to the left of the SMA and SMV can sometimes present a diagnostic challenge. Patients may complain of vague, poorly localized upper abdominal pain or dyspepsia. The differential diagnosis for tumors to the left of the SMA

TABLE 9.2. Selected series on the surgical management of nonfunctioning pancreatic endocrine tumors (PETs).

| Author (year) | No. of patients with | | Synchronous liver metastases | Overall survival | Study years |
|---|---|---|---|---|---|
| | PETs (NFT) | Curative resection of primary (metastases) | | | |
| Legaspi et al. (1988) | 33 (22) | 11 (0) | 16 | 76% at 3 years | 1983–1988 |
| Thompson et al. (1988) | 58 (27) | 15 (0) | 19 | 42% at 5 years | 1965–1984 |
| Kim et al. (1988) | 20 (13) | 6 (0) | 14 | NA | 1974–1988 |
| McEntee et al. (1990) | 13 (3) | 2[a] (6) | 13 | NA | 1970–1989 |
| Carty et al. (1992) | 17 (0) | 14 (13) | 17 | 79% at 5 years | 1982–1991 |
| Evans et al. (1993) | 73 (73) | 19 (0) | 34 | 5 years (median) | 1953–1992 |
| Udelsman et al. (1993) | 12 (4) | 11 (1) | 2 | 92% at 3.5 years | 1982–1991 |
| Cheslin-Curtis et al. (1993) | 20 (20) | 12 (2) | 5 | 30 m (median) | 1982–1991 |
| Lo et al. (1996) | 64 (34) | 17 (0) | 39 | 49% at 5 years | 1985–1993 |
| Madura et al. (1997) | 14 (14) | 13 (0) | 0 | 31 m (median) | 1988–1996 |
| Madeira et al. (1998) | 82 (44) | 35 (5) | 49 | NA | 1991–1997 |
| Bartsch et al. (1999) | 18 (18) | 11 (1) | 3 | 65% at 5 years | 1983–1998 |

(continued)

TABLE 9.2. (continued).

| Author (year) | No. of patients with | | Synchronous liver metastases | Overall survival | Study years |
|---|---|---|---|---|---|
| | PETs (NFT) | Curative resection of primary (metastases) | | | |
| Solorzano et al. (2001) | 163 (163) | 42 (4) | 101 | 3.2 years (median) or 43% at 5 years | 1988–1999 |
| Sarmiento et al. (2002) | 23 (7) | 9 (9) | 23 | 76 m (median) or 71% at 5 years | 1980–1998 |
| Gullo et al. (2003) | 184 (184) | 124 (0) | 69[b] | NA | 1987–2001 |
| Elias et al. (2003) | 23 (23) | 15[a] (23) | 23 | 71% at 5 years | 1985–2000 |
| Pape et al. (2004) | 73 (50) | NA | 53[b] | 47 m (median) or 42.9 at 5 years | 1980–2002 |
| Liang et al. (2004) | 28 (28) | 17 (0) | 6 | 60 m (median) or 58% at 5 years | 1972–2002 |

TABLE 9.3. Differential diagnosis for tumors to the left of the superior mesenteric artery and superior mesenteric vein.

| Organ or site of origin | Pathology |
| --- | --- |
| Adrenal | Adrenocortical carcinoma |
| | Adenoma |
| | Pheochromocytoma |
| Colon | Splenic flexure adenocarcinoma |
| Retroperitoneum | Sarcoma |
| Kidney | Renal cell carcinoma |
| Stomach | Gastrointestinal stromal tumor |
| Pancreas | Pancreatic endocrine tumor |
| | Adenocarcinoma |
| | Cystic pancreatic tumor |

and SMV is listed in > Table 9.3. Serum PP, CgA, glucagon, VIP, and CA 19-9 levels should be obtained. Upper and lower gastrointestinal endoscopy should be used to rule out gastric and colonic tumors. Lastly, functional adrenal tumors should be excluded by obtaining a plasma cortisol and metanephrine level. Tumors of the stomach (gastrointestinal stromal tumors), colon (locally advanced adenocarcinoma), adrenal gland (adrenocortical carcinoma, pheochromocytoma), and kidney (renal cell carcinoma) can be confused with PETs, especially if peptide production is subtle or absent. Radiographic evaluation and biochemical screening can aid in making the correct diagnosis. In patients with sporadic nonfunctioning PET, surgical resection is the preferred treatment if technically possible.

## Operative Management and Outcome

The goals of operative resection of nonfunctioning PETs are to improve local disease control and to increase quality and length of patient survival. Therefore, the potential operative morbidity and complications of insulin dependence and gastrointestinal dysfunction need to be considered when planning operative intervention. Previous reports have demonstrated that resection of a primary tumor in the presence of metastatic disease does not prolong patient survival.

Five-year overall survival for nonfunctioning PETs has been reported to range from 42% to 71% (median, 2.5–5 years) (Table 9.2). In a large single institution series of 163 patients with nonfunctioning PETs, patients with metastatic disease at the time of diagnosis had a median survival of 2.2 years compared to 7.1 years for patients with localized, non-metastatic disease ($p < 0.0001$). Although nonfunctioning PETs are believed to have an indolent course and better tumor biology when compared to adenocarcinoma of the pancreas, it is important to note that the majority of patients in this series died of metastatic PET. Further, only 42 (26%) of the 163 patients were able to have a potentially curative resection of their primary tumor. Survival advantage was demonstrated for patients who underwent complete resection of the primary tumor in the absence of metastatic disease. However, only 20 (48%) of the 42 patients who underwent resection of the primary tumor were alive without evidence of recurrent disease at last follow-up. Based upon these data, it is inappropriate to assume that complete resection of the primary tumor in the absence of metastatic disease corresponds to a long-term cure. Of 20 patients in this large series who had locally advanced primary tumors in the absence of metastatic disease, 12 (60%) died of disease. Ten of these 12 patients had tumors in the head of the pancreas. Prior to death, these 10 patients had a median of 2 hospital admissions each for complications related to their primary tumor process or attempts to treat that tumor process: biliary obstruction, gastric outlet obstruction, gastrointestinal hemorrhage, or treatment-related toxicity. These data demonstrate that primary tumors to the right of the superior mesenteric vessels are associated with substantial patient morbidity and are best managed by pancreaticoduodenectomy, occasionally requiring in continuity vascular or adjacent organ resection for adequate local-regional control.

The median survival in this series for patients presenting with hepatic metastatic disease ranged from 1.8 to 3 years. Although the duration of survival of patients with metastatic nonfunctioning PET is clearly superior to that of patients with metastatic adenocarcinoma of the pancreas, the majority of patients with metastatic nonfunctioning PET will die of disease within 2 years of diagnosis. Therefore, both regional and systemic therapies and investigational protocol-based treatments should be considered at the time of diagnosis in these patients. Furthermore, the difference in survival duration in this series between patients with hepatic metastatic disease who either did or did not undergo resection of their primary tumor, did not achieve statistical significance despite the inherent selection bias in favor of those who underwent resection of the primary tumor. Those who underwent resection of the primary tumor were those most likely to have less extensive extrapancreatic disease and a better performance status.

Body and tail nonfunctioning PETs rarely cause symptoms and are often locally advanced or metastatic at diagnosis. Patients with liver metastases from primary PETs in the body and tail achieved no benefit from distal pancreatectomy in the absence of symptoms related to the primary tumor. Therefore, if the primary is asymptomatic, there is little role for pancreatectomy in treating nonfunctioning PETs of the body or tail in the presence of unresectable extrapancreatic metastatic disease. This concept may change as strategies for the management of hepatic metastases become more successful.

There may be a place for pancreaticoduodenectomy in selected good-risk patients with nonfunctioning PET of the pancreatic head who have low-volume extrapancreatic metastatic disease. Tumors of the pancreatic head, in contrast to tumors of the distal pancreas, may erode into the duodenum, resulting in gastrointestinal hemorrhage, or may cause biliary or gastric outlet obstruction. Such complications are better managed with resection of the primary tumor rather than palliative bypass procedures. Lastly, despite anecdotal reports of successful combined curative resection of the primary tumor and hepatic metastases, such an aggressive surgical approach is only possible in a selected few (Table 9.2). Most of these patients present with bilobar metastases that are not amenable to curative resection.

A treatment algorithm for the patient with a sporadic nonfunctioning PET is outlined in Fig. 9.2. In the presence of hepatic metastases, consideration of resection of the primary tumor is given only in patients with good performance status and low volume metastatic disease. For example: A young patient who presents with biliary obstruction due to a PET in the pancreatic head. At laparotomy, multiple 1 cm nodules are seen in the liver, and biopsy confirms metastatic PET. This patient has a high probability of incurring major morbidity due to uncontrolled growth of the primary tumor prior to death from metastatic disease, and would benefit from resection of the primary tumor.

In a recent report and review of the worldwide literature, Assalia and Gagner concluded that laparoscopic resection for solitary, benign PETs, mainly insulinomas in the body and tail of the pancreas duplicates the success of conventional surgery with regards to localization and cure of disease. The main morbidity was the 18% incidence of pancreatic fistula.

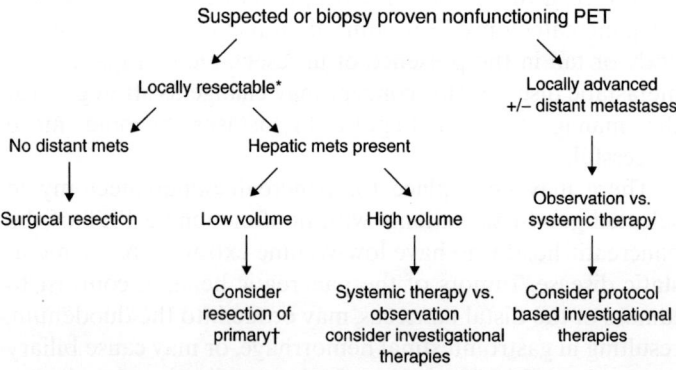

FIGURE 9.2. Strategy for treatment of a patient presenting with suspected or biopsy-proven nonfunctioning PET. *No encasement of SMA or celiac axis, patent SMV-portal vein confluence. †In selected cases as discussed in text.

Only 7 of the 93 patients had nonfunctioning PETs. Further study is needed to evaluate the role of laparoscopy in the treatment of nonfunctioning PETs.

With the increased use of radiographic studies to evaluate other conditions, there has been an increase in the incidental diagnosis of small (1–2 cm) asymptomatic nonfunctioning sporadic PETs. We believe that formal pancreatic resection should be carried out whenever possible. An exception would be a small lesion in the head of the pancreas that would require a pancreaticoduodenectomy, especially if the patient is a poor risk because of medical comorbidities.

## Extended Resection

Occasionally, nonfunctioning PET will require an extended operation to achieve a complete resection. The technical limitations to successful resection in these patients are arterial encasement (SMA, hepatic artery (HA), or celiac axis), venous encasement, or occlusion (SMPV confluence). Several investigators have demonstrated the safety of segmental resection of the SMPV confluence when necessary to allow complete resection. Resection of the SMA is associated with high morbidity and mortality; therefore we continue to consider it a contraindication to surgical resection of a nonfunctioning PET.

Locally advanced tumors of the upper portion of the head and neck of the pancreas may encase the celiac axis or HA without involving the SMA. If the left gastric artery is not involved, the stomach can be preserved. Typically, large tumors of the neck and body of the pancreas involve the HA and the left gastric and splenic arteries near their origin, and tumor extirpation requires upper abdominal exenteration with removal of the stomach and spleen, in addition to total pancreaticoduodenectomy. The combination of total pancreaticoduodenectomy plus total gastrectomy leads to long-term gastrointestinal dysfunction, especially when combined with an extensive retroperitoneal dissection with removal of the celiac and mesenteric neural plexus. For these reasons, such resections should be reserved for highly selected patients and only performed when complete tumor extirpation appears possible based on preoperative imaging studies. Because the median survival can be as high as 5 years in patients with unresected nonmetastatic nonfunctioning PET, it becomes difficult to recommend operation as the complexity and potential morbidity of the surgical procedure increases. With further advances in operative technique and nutritional support, the extent of surgical resection advisable in patients with non-metastatic nonfunctioning PETs may increase.

## Treatment of Locally Advanced Disease

The appropriate management of locally advanced, surgically unresectable PETs in patients without extrapancreatic metastatic disease remains debatable. Operative treatment is often necessary to palliate biliary and/or gastric outlet obstruction and may be more durable than less invasive endoscopic techniques. For oncologic treatment, cytotoxic chemotherapy is considered when there is radiographic evidence of disease progression or symptoms develop. Octreotide or interferon-alpha can result in disease stabilization; however, these therapies rarely result in a radiographically definable response. No data exist to support the use of adjuvant chemo-radiotherapy in patients with PET. The experience with radiation therapy for locally advanced pancreatic neuroendocrine carcinoma is anecdotal.

## Men-1

The surgical management of PETs in the setting of MEN-1 is controversial. In these patients, the entire pancreas is at risk to develop a PET and multiple tumors are the rule. The standard goal of operation in patients with MEN-1 is to relieve the symptoms of hormonal excess (insulin, gastrin) and to prevent the development of liver metastases. Currently, there is no clear relationship between specific *MEN1* gene mutations and the phenotypic manifestations of the disease. There is no reliable way of monitoring the propensity of these tumors to develop liver metastases. The only way to potentially prevent the development of liver metastases in patients with MEN-1 who develop a pancreatic neoplasm (functioning or nonfunctioning) would be to perform a total pancreaticoduodenectomy. This procedure invariably leads to long-term metabolic complications. Ideally, one would remove only identifiable tumor and leave enough pancreas to preserve endocrine and exocrine function.

Because of the multiplicity of the PETs in patients with MEN-1, as well as low rates of clinical cure, some investigators have discouraged early operative intervention in MEN-1 patients with PETs. In 1999, Norton and associates reported the National Cancer Institute (NCI) experience with surgical treatment of the Zollinger-Ellison syndrome. There were 28 patients with MEN-1. All MEN-1 patients had relatively large tumors (3 cm or greater) by the time they had their operation. No patient with MEN-1 was free of disease at 10 years.

On the other hand, Thompson and co-investigators at the University of Michigan have recommended a more aggressive approach; they consider exploration of patients with only biochemical evidence for disease. Since size is not a reliable predictor of malignant behavior and metastatic disease may be present in MEN-1 patients even when the primary tumors are small, Thompson and others have recommended that pancreatic tumors of any size identified on preoperative imaging (CT and endoscopic ultrasound) be considered for operation. Patients with MEN-1 and biochemical evidence for gastrinoma without imaging evidence for disease may also be considered for operation with or without regionalization of their tumors by intra-arterial secretin stimulation of gastrin. A standard operative approach in patients with hypergastrinemia is taken, with full mobilization of the pancreas, use of intraoperative ultrasound, resection of pancreatic body and tail tumors by a distal subtotal pancreatectomy,

enucleation of tumors in the pancreatic head, a portal peripancreatic and periduodenal lymph node dissection, and a
duodenotomy with palpation of the duodenal wall and resection of any identified tumors. This aggressive surgical approach
in 11 MEN-1 patients with gastrinoma resulted in normal
serum gastrin levels in 10 of 11 patients after follow-up ranging from 3 months to 14 years. Kouvaraki and colleagues
retrospectively evaluated the impact that surgical treatment
of the primary tumor would have on the development of liver
metastases in 55 patients with MEN-1. This study demonstrated that surgical excision of MEN-1 related PETs in
young patients with localized tumors at diagnosis improved
survival. Although there is no prospective proof of benefit of
resection in these patients, an aggressive approach as described
above is reasonable in selected patients, particularly those
with hypergastrinemia who are from MEN-1 kindreds in
whom there is a history of malignant PETs with hepatic
metastasis, as well as any good-risk MEN-1 patient with pancreatic tumors identified on imaging studies.

## Medical Directed Therapies

If the primary tumor is not symptomatic, pancreatic resection
in the presence of unresectable extra-pancreatic metastatic
disease is not indicated. Aggressive management of the primary tumor despite the presence of extrapancreatic disease
may be more compelling as treatments for metastatic disease
become more effective. Systemic chemotherapy, biological
therapies, molecular targeted therapies, radiopharmaceuti-
cals, hepatic artery embolization, radiofrequency ablation,
cryotherapy, and liver transplantation remain areas of investigation that may ultimately change stage-specific treatment
recommendations.

The primary chemotherapeutic agent used in nonfunctioning PETs is streptozotocin. Combination therapy of streptozotocin with 5-FU is associated with improved response rates
and survival duration. Moertel, et al. conducted a multicenter
clinical trial in patients with advanced islet cell carcinoma

and demonstrated that the combination of streptozocin with doxorubicin was associated with the best response rates and duration of response when compared to streptozocin plus 5-FU or chlorozotocin alone. The combination of 5-FU, doxorubicin, and streptozotocin (FAS) has also been investigated with good results. Chemotherapy is usually considered in patients with unresectable locally advanced or metastatic PETs who have local symptoms and/or progression of their disease. Molecular targeted therapies against epidermal growth factor receptor (Gefitnib) and vascular endothelial growth factor (SU-11248) in pancreatic islet cell and carcinoid tumors are under active investigation.

Neuroendocrine tumors including PETs have somatostatin receptors. Somatostatin receptors mediate growth and secretion of peptide hormones in these tumors. The somatostatin analog, octreotide can control peptide secretion from functioning PETs and may halt PET growth, but rarely results in objective tumor responses. Interferon-alpha alone or in combination with octreotide has led to symptomatic control, biochemical responses, and/or tumoristatic effects when used to treat PETs. Unfortunately, like octreotide, objective tumor responses to interferon have been disappointing.

## Treatment of Liver Metastases

Multiple retrospective reports have documented the safety of hepatic resection, cryosurgical ablation, and radiofrequency ablation (RFA) in selected patients with PET metastatic to the liver. The effect on survival of an aggressive approach in patients with metastatic nonfunctional PET remains unproven. For now, these approaches are reasonable in selected patients with relatively low-volume and slow-growing disease confined to the liver.

Hepatic artery embolization or chemoembolization may be considered in patients with hepatic metastases from nonfunctioning PET. This approach may be favored in patients not considered candidates for surgical resection or ablative therapies due to the extent of liver involvement. Isolation perfusion of the liver for hepatic metastases from PET, as performed at the NCI, remains an investigational procedure.

Liver transplantation may be justified in a selected subset of symptomatic patients with metastatic neuroendocrine carcinoma confined to the liver. In the United States, limitations on the availability of livers for transplantation and the good performance status of most patients with metastatic PET, results in a situation in which these patients are too low on transplant priority lists to be considered active candidates until their cancer has progressed to the point that they are effectively excluded.

## Conclusions

Patients with nonfunctioning PETs have relatively long survival compared with patients with adenocarcinoma of the pancreas; but the majority of patients who do not undergo a potentially curative resection die of their disease less than 5 years after diagnosis. The decision to proceed with operative resection of the primary pancreatic tumor should be based on its location in the pancreas, the extent of resection required, and the presence or absence of metastatic disease. Systemic therapy and regional therapies, along with investigational protocol-based treatments, should be considered for patients with a good performance status who have locally advanced primary tumors or metastatic disease.

## Selected Readings

Alexander HR, Jensen RT (2005) Pancreatic endocrine tumors. In: DeVita VT Jr, Hellman S, Rosenberg SA (eds) Cancer principles and practice of oncology, 7th edn. Lippincott, Williams & Wilkins, Philadelphia, pp 1540–1558

Cheslyn-Curtis S, Sitaram V, Williamson RC (1993) Management of non-functioning neuroendocrine tumours of the pancreas. Br J Surg 80:625–627

Evans DB, Skibber JM, Lee JE, et al. (1993) Nonfunctioning islet cell carcinoma of the pancreas. Surgery 114:1175–1181

Gullo L, Migliori M, Falconi M, et al. (2003) Nonfunctioning pancreatic endocrine tumors: a multicenter clinical study. Gut 98:2435–2439

Kouvaraki MA, Shapiro SE, Cote GJ, et al. (2006) Management of pancreatic endocrine tumors in multiple endocrine neoplasia type 1. World J Surg 30:643–653

Kouvaraki MA, Solorzano CC, Shapiro SE, et al. (2005) Surgical treatment of non-functioning pancreatic islet cell tumors. J Surg Oncol 89:170–185

Sarmiento JM, Que FG, Grant CS, et al. (2002) Concurrent resections of pancreatic islet cell cancers with synchronous hepatic metastases: outcomes of an aggressive approach. Surgery 132:976–982

Solorzano CC, Lee JE, Pisters PWT, et al. (2001) Nonfunctioning islet cell carcinoma of the pancreas: survival results in a contemporary series of 163 patients. Surgery 130:1078–1085

Solorzano CC, Lee JE (2005) Nonfunctioning pancreatic endocrine tumors. In: Von Hoff DD, Evans DB, Hruban RH (eds) Pancreatic cancer. Jones & Bartlett, Boston, MA, pp 663–676

Thompson GB, van Heerden JA, Grant CS, et al. (1988) Islet cell carcinomas of the pancreas: a twenty-year experience. Surgery 104:1011–1017

Wiedenmann B, Jensen RT, Mignon M, et al. (1998) Preoperative diagnosis and surgical management of neuroendocrine gastroenteropancreatic tumors: general recommendations by a consensus workshop. World J Surg 22:309–318

# Part III
# Spleen — Benign

# 10
# Splenectomy

**Robert T. A. Padbury**

## Pearls and Pitfalls

- Aim to preserve splenic tissue whenever possible.
- Partial splenectomy and splenorrhaphy are valuable techniques to achieve functional splenic preservation.
- In case of total splenectomy for trauma, splenic autotransplantation should be considered.
- Nonoperative management of splenic trauma is very successful in appropriately selected patients.
- Delayed splenic rupture is uncommon after 2 weeks.
- Morbidity and mortality is significantly greater for splenectomy in myelofibrosis and malignant hematologic conditions.
- Overwhelming postsplenectomy sepsis (OPSI) remains a lifelong risk in asplenic patients, especially in children.
- Immunization against polysaccharide-encapsulated bacteria (pneumococcus, meningococcus, and *Hemophilus influenza*) should be administered at least 2 weeks prior to splenectomy or 2 weeks after emergency splenectomy.
- Signs of infection should be treated rapidly in asplenic patients.

K.I. Bland et al. (eds.), *Surgery of the Pancreas and Spleen*, DOI: 10.1007/978-1-84996-369-5_10,
© Springer-Verlag London Limited 2011

# Indications for Splenectomy

Elective splenectomy is performed either to alter the course of a disease involving the spleen or to provide symptomatic relief from the physical effects of splenic enlargement or the clinical effects of hypersplenism (Table 10.1). In contrast, emergency splenectomy occurs in the setting of trauma.

Splenectomy may be undertaken via an open or laparoscopic approach. Further, the splenectomy may be total or partial, and in cases of trauma, splenic repair or splenorrhaphy can often be successful in preserving functional splenic tissue. As the long-term consequences of splenectomy were better understood, clinical determination to preserve splenic tissue has evolved. This appreciation of the role of the spleen and the type of splenic tissue necessary to maintain function has led over time to fewer splenectomies and a greater proportion of partial resections. The laparoscopic approach has evolved over the last 15 years, and larger and more difficult resections are undertaken with minimal access techniques.

In this chapter the indications for splenectomy and the long-term outcomes are described, concentrating on the adult population. For details of operative techniques for the various approaches to splenectomy and splenic repair, see Clavien et al. (2008).

## Trauma

The evolution of splenic preservation has been reflected in the approach to patients with splenic trauma. The clinical management to achieve splenic preservation continues to evolve. A few decades ago, splenectomy was performed invariably in trauma laparotomies, even if the organ had stopped bleeding at the time of operation. In the late 1970s and 1980s, splenorrhaphy was developed and was applied widely where possible.

With increasing accuracy and availability of abdominal computed tomography (CT), the requirement to undertake laparotomy to diagnose associated abdominal injuries

TABLE 10.1. Indications for splenectomy

| Trauma |
|---|
| Incidental |
|   Operative injury |
|   Included with disease removal eg., distal pancreas tumor |
| Splenic artery aneurysm |
| Splenic cyst |
|   Parasitic |
|   Nonparasitic |
| Splenic abscess |
| Idiopathic thrombocytopenic purpura (ITP) |
| Hereditary spherocytosis |
| Autoimmune hemolytic anemia |
| Felty's syndrome |
| Myelofibrosis |
| Refractory anemia (myelodysplasia) |
| Plasma cell dyscrasias |
| "Idiopathic" splenomegaly |
| Hematologic malignancy |
|   Hodgkin's lymphoma |
|   Non-Hodgkin's lymphoma |
|   Chronic lymphatic leukemia |
|   Chronic myeloid leukemia |
|   Plasma cell myeloma |

declined. This noninvasive imaging modality, coupled with the observation that once the spleen stopped bleeding, further hemorrhage was relatively infrequent, resulted in the widespread adoption of nonoperative observational management of splenic trauma in patients with hemodynamic stability and an absence of other injuries requiring operative treatment.

The indication for early splenectomy in the trauma setting is initial hemodynamic instability as a result of the splenic trauma. Splenorrhaphy or partial splenectomy may be undertaken if the circumstances allow. If there are substantive coexistent injuries, effective and safe control of the patient may require rapid total splenectomy.

Nonoperative management of traumatic splenic injuries is successful in more than 90% of appropriately selected patients. Indications for operative intervention in patients selected initially for nonoperative management include large accumulation of intra-abdominal blood, more than two units of blood transfused for the splenic injury, a decreasing hemoglobin level, or the development of hemodynamic instability. In the situation of rescue surgery of nonoperative management, splenorrhaphy or partial splenectomy can be considered. There is a greater failure rate of nonoperative management in older patients and those with multiple severe injuries. Nonoperative management is less likely to be successful with higher CT grades of splenic injury; usually, these higher grade injuries are associated with hemodynamic instability, and the decision to operate is made on clinical grounds rather than CT criteria.

The outcomes of splenectomy for trauma are generally very good with early mortality specific to the splenectomy of <1%. Most of the mortality is related to associated injuries, often extra-abdominal.

*Delayed rupture of the spleen*. The major clinical concern with nonoperative management of splenic trauma is delayed rupture, particularly in patients after discharge from the hospital. Most cases of delayed rupture occur within the first 7 or 8 days. Delayed rupture is rare after 2 weeks. Late splenic abscess formation has been reported and may be an indication for late splenectomy.

Follow-up CT evaluation is not required routinely. CT evaluation is recommended, however, for higher-risk patients, such as those with large hematomas, with grade IV injuries with hilar vessel involvement, or with contrast blush on the initial CT (see also "Return to contact sports" below).

*Return to contact sports.* A further question after recovery of patients with the nonoperative management of splenic trauma is time to return to contact sports. Experimental evidence indicates that splenic lacerations repair with a tensile strength equal to, or greater than, normal splenic tissue within 6 weeks. Follow-up imaging studies of human subjects with splenic hematomas indicate that the time to healing or linear scar formation varies with the grade of injury. Lacerations will heal within 3–6 weeks (as per the experimental evidence), but larger splenic hematomas will take a longer period of time, up to 12–16 weeks. There are no good clinical data on the safety of return to contact sports, but for splenic lacerations, a minimum 6 weeks off seems appropriate, and for large hematomas, documentation of healing with linear scar formation would seem appropriate prior to return to active participation.

## Incidental Splenectomy

*Operative injury.* Estimates of inadvertent iatrogenic splenic injury from the USA and elsewhere suggest that intraoperative injury during fundoplication, distal pancreatectomy, colectomy, or left nephrectomy is a common indication for splenectomy. In the current era, splenic hemorrhage in this situation should be readily amenable to splenorrhaphy or partial splenectomy, even if it requires summoning to the operating theater a surgeon with more experience in these techniques.

*Removal of adjacent or extensive neoplasms.* Large neoplasms or other masses in the tail of the pancreas, gastric neoplasms, and some other neoplasms in the upper abdomen may require splenectomy for surgical clearance. Ideally, the need for splenectomy should be predictable before the operation is undertaken and immunizations administered at least 2 weeks prior (see "OPSI" below).

# Splenic Artery Aneurysm

Splenic artery aneurysms and pseudoaneurysms are often managed via percutaneous techniques and angiographic embolization. If unsuccessful, laparoscopic or open intervention to ligate and/or remove the diseased artery is necessary. Provided the spleen is not fully mobilized, it will usually survive ligation of the splenic artery and therefore can be spared. In cases of aneurysm rupture, splenectomy is usually required.

# Splenic Cysts

*Parasitic cysts.* Worldwide, parasitic splenic cysts are far more common than nonparasitic cystic lesions. Hydatid disease (echinococcosis) is by far the most common parasitic cyst of the spleen. Care must be taken during the operation not to rupture the cyst and spread the parasite throughout the peritoneal cavity. Operative intervention involves resection of the cyst, if possible, with either total or partial splenectomy. Marsupialization and evacuation of cyst contents is an alternative if splenectomy is too difficult or hazardous.

*Nonparasitic cysts.* This is a rare clinical entity. The cysts are either primary or secondary (pseudocysts resulting from liquefaction of old hematoma – yet more than 50% of patients are unable to recall a significant traumatic event). Operative intervention is required for large (>5 cm) symptomatic or complicated cysts. Aspiration and attempted sclerosis of cysts are generally ineffective. Surgical options include total or partial splenectomy or cyst de-roofing performed either laparoscopically or open. Recurrence after de-roofing is relatively frequent, and resection is most appropriate if possible. Malignancy in splenic cysts is very rare, and overall, partial splenectomy appears the best option; recurrence has not been described, and the whole cyst is available for histologic analysis.

# Splenic Abscess

Splenic abscess is encountered rarely but may be associated with bacterial endocarditis, intravenous drug addiction, or infection of a splenic hematoma or area of infarction. It is also more common in the immunosuppressed. Percutaneous drainage and antibiotics are often successful in single, isolated splenic abscesses, but splenectomy may be required, especially with multiple splenic abscesses.

# Idiopathic Thrombocytopenic Purpura

Idiopathic thrombocytopenic purpura (ITP) in adulthood is often refractory to steroid withdrawal and may require splenectomy. It is characterized by a low platelet count, hemorrhagic tendencies, and a normal bone marrow biopsy. Being the site of production of the antiplatelet antibodies, the spleen is a major site of destruction of the sensitized platelets.

Indications for splenectomy in this condition include recurrent thrombocytopenia on steroid withdrawal or tapering, a persistently required daily dose of prednisolone >10 mg, or signs of hemorrhage despite maximum medical therapy. Generally, all patients with a platelet count $<10 \times 10^9/l$ and those patients with a moderate or worse bleeding tendency and a platelet count between $10 \times 10^9/l$ and $30 \times 30^9/l$ will require splenectomy. In order of importance in recommending splenectomy is (a) bleeding tendency, (b) drug requirements to control bleeding and finally (c) the absolute platelet count.

No reliable or clinically valuable indicators are prognostic of a good, durable response to splenectomy. Platelet counts will usually increase to near normal levels within a week. Approximately 75% of patients with ITP will require a splenectomy ultimately, and a good moderate term result will occur in 75% of these. Failures generally occur within 2 years, but late, long-term failures do occur, giving around 65% long-term overall success.

Because about 15% of individuals have an accessory spleen, it is important that a thorough search for these often hidden accessory spleens is undertaken. In patients who relapse, a proportion will be found to have an accessory spleen, the identification and removal of which can lead to a good secondary result.

Splenectomy for ITP is very well suited to the laparoscopic approach. Results are very similar in thrombocytopenia associated with systemic lupus erythematous (SLE), which is also immune-mediated.

# Thrombotic Thrombocytopenic Purpura (TTP)

This rare condition is characterized by microcirculatory occlusion from platelet aggregates. The clinical manifestations are fever, renal failure, and neurologic sequelae. Plasma exchange remains the standard therapy, but splenectomy is indicated for refractory cases. Response is unpredictable, but favorable outcomes can be expected in over 50%.

# Hereditary Spherocytosis

This rare, autosomal dominant condition involves a defect in the red blood cell membrane leading to abnormal morphology and a shorter life span of the circulating red blood cells. Clinical features are generally those of chronic hemolysis with anemia, mild jaundice, splenomegaly, and gallstones (bilirubinate stones secondary to chronic hemolysis). Splenectomy may be required for severe or moderate forms. Splenectomy (and cholecystectomy!) is performed generally in childhood but may be extended to young adulthood.

The aim of splenectomy is to treat anemia, gallstones, aplastic crises, and late hemochromatosis.

The primary indication for operation may actually be gallstones, and at the time of the gallbladder surgery, splenectomy is recommended. Conversely, if splenectomy is indicated for another reason (e.g., anemia), gallstones should be sought, and, if found, a cholecystectomy undertaken. Splenomegaly alone is not an indication for splenectomy in this condition. After splenectomy, red blood cell survival returns to very near normal despite bizarre cell morphology on the postsplenectomy film.

## Autoimmune Hemolytic Anemia

This spectrum of disorders is characterized by hemolysis with anemia and reticulocytosis, intermittent jaundice, and splenomegaly. The variant with warm reactive antibodies is associated with sequestration and destruction of red blood cells in the spleen. Steroids are the first line of therapy, but if unsuccessful, splenectomy is indicated. A sustained response occurs in approximately 70%.

## Felty's Syndrome

The triad of severe rheumatoid arthritis, granulocytopenia, and splenomegaly constitute Felty's syndrome. Severe, recurrent infections are characteristic of this disorder with an absence of neutrophilia. Splenectomy is effective in individuals with significant recurrent infections and chronic leg ulcers. Long-term correction of the granulocyte count is achieved in approximately 80%, and up to 50% will not have any further infections.

## Myelofibrosis

Indications for splenectomy in this condition are related to the symptomatology of the huge splenomegaly from mechanical symptoms (size, splenic infarction, pain); in contrast, portal hypertension, anemia, and thrombocytopenia are not the drivers to consider splenectomy. A palliative benefit is anticipated in 70%.

Unlike most other conditions leading to consideration of elective splenectomy, in myelofibrosis, the splenectomy itself is associated with a very real morbidity (~30%) and mortality (15%). Therefore, when splenectomy is being considered, extremely honest, realistic discussion with the family and patient is imperative. Complications and mortality are much more common after splenectomy for this indication. Specific early complications that occur with higher frequency in this disorder include postoperative hemorrhage and thrombosis. Postoperative bleeding is often from the diaphragmatic surface, and very close attention to hemostasis, particularly in this area, is essential. Careful monitoring of postoperative thrombocytosis in this condition is also recommended; some surgeons suggest routine scanning of splanchnic vessels with Doppler ultrasonography in an attempt to detect thrombosis in the splanchnic venous system. Anticoagulation should be instituted if evidence of thrombus is identified. A number of thrombo-hemorrhagic events can occur in even patients with relatively normal platelet counts.

In the longer term, accelerated hepatomegaly (hepatic sequestration of myeloid elements) and leukemic transformation (15%) complicate the clinical course. Survival after splenectomy is guarded, with 25% of patients succumbing within 6 months. Two thirds survive beyond 12 months. It must be acknowledged with patient and family that survival is not influenced by the indication for surgery.

Patients with refractory anemia due to myelodysplasia with increasing transfusion requirements associated with increased splenic activity may have their transfusion requirements decreased substantially after splenectomy. Patients must be selected carefully, because many are elderly with clinically important comorbidities, but quality of life can be improved in those who respond.

## Plasma Cell Dyscrasias

This group of disorders is characterized by a proliferation of B cells and production of a monoclonal immunoglobulin or polypeptide. Examples include Waldenstrom's macroglobulinemia and primary amyloidosis. Indications for splenectomy include hypersplenism and hemolytic anemia, massive splenomegaly, splenic rupture (particularly in primary amyloidosis) and very rarely splenic plasmacytomas.

# Diagnostic Splenectomy for "Idiopathic" Splenomegaly

There is a clinical scenario characterized by splenomegaly, usually with symptoms and varying degrees of cytopenia, occurring in patients in whom bone marrow aspiration and other investigations are inconclusive. With our increasing understanding of hematologic disorders, the number of these cases is now small, but splenectomy will facilitate diagnosis and in some cases be therapeutic. Diagnosis is often one of a questionable hematologic malignancy, but other conditions, such as sarcoidosis, Castleman's disease, and congestive splenomegaly secondary to portal hypertension, will be found.

# Hematological Malignancy

Splenectomy for hematologic malignancy (as with myelofibrosis) is generally more difficult and is associated with a higher mortality, morbidity, and a conversion rate when attempted laparoscopically. Splenectomy may be indicated to relieve features of hypersplenism, to decrease transfusion requirements, for mechanical symptoms, and occasionally for staging or to establish a tissue diagnosis.

*Hodgkin's lymphoma.* Prior to the 1980s, staging splenectomy was a common component of the diagnostic workup. Staging laparotomy and splenectomy is now uncommon but may be indicated when a negative result will allow withholding of chemotherapy. Surgery may be indicated when a negative result will allow withholding of chemotherapy, i.e., in true stage 1 disease when radiotherapy may be curative.

*Non-Hodgkin's lymphoma.* Splenectomy may be undertaken for diagnostic or therapeutic reasons. Correction of cytopenias and symptoms of splenic enlargement are the current indications. Splenectomy may also be required for diagnosis and facilitation for chemotherapy.

*Chronic myeloid leukemia.* Survival is not improved by splenectomy, and there is an increase in thromboembolism and vascular complications compared with patients with CML not undergoing splenectomy. Therefore, as with myelofibrosis, consideration of splenectomy for symptomatic reasons should be carefully discussed and reconsidered. The modern use of highly effective kinase inhibitors means that gross organomegaly is no longer a continuing problem in this group of patients.

*Chronic lymphatic leukemia.* Indications for splenectomy include hypersplenism and symptomatic splenomegaly. Marked improvements in hemoglobin and platelet count may occur. Hairy cell leukemia is a rare variant of chronic lymphocystic leukemia (CLL), for which a splenectomy was once a usual part of management. It is now required rarely because of improvements in chemotherapy.

# Complications and Postoperative Management

The early and late complications of splenectomy are listed in Table 10.2. Postoperative management after splenectomy is usually standard as for other intra-abdominal surgery. There is no apparent benefit for postoperative nasogastric decompression or intraperitoneal drain. If either is used, early removal is recommended.

There is no evidence that routine monitoring of the platelet count and institution of anticoagulation is indicated for most conditions, except in patients with myelofibrosis and hematologic malignancy. Patients with these diseases are at much greater risk of splanchnic thrombosis; postoperative abdominal pain and fever should be investigated aggressively with Doppler ultrasonography (see section on "Myelofibrosis").

Intraoperative rupture should be carefully avoided when the indication for splenectomy is nonmalignant hematologic

TABLE 10.2. Complications of splenectomy

**Early**

Intraoperative rupture

Failure to detect accessory spleen

Postoperative hemorrhage

Infections

   Subphrenic abscess

   Wound

Pulmonary

   Pulmonary embolus

   Pneumonia

   Pneumorothorax

   Atelectasis

Intestinal

   Delayed gastric emptying

   Gastric leak/fistula

Pancreas

   Pancreatitis

   Pancreatic fistula

   Pancreatic pseudocyst

Thromboembolic

   Splanchnic ischemia

**Long-term**

OPSI

Ischemic heart disease

   (Thromboembolic: no increased risk)

   (Cancer: no increased risk)

disorder. Similarly, accessory spleens should be sought, identified, and removed.

In the long term, the major risk is OPSI. A full description is given below. There is possibly an increase in the death rate from myocardial ischemia, but no apparent increase in the risk of long-term thromboembolic phenomena. There is no increase in the risk of developing non-hematologic cancer.

## Overwhelming Postsplenectomy Infection

The phenomenon of OPSI was first suggested experimentally in the early 1900s and first reported in infants in 1952. Subsequent observations have confirmed the susceptibility, albeit decreased, in adults.

The risk of OPSI in adults may not be as high as in children under 6, but when OPSI occurs, the mortality rate approaches 50%. Death can ensue within hours of the first symptoms.

The risk is least in patients undergoing splenectomy for trauma, intermediate after splenectomy for benign hematologic conditions, and greatest in those with reticuloendothelial disease or hematologic malignancy, especially in children.

The risk of overwhelming sepsis is around 60 times greater than normal. Patients are particularly at risk from sepsis from encapsulated organisms, which has resulted in immunization against the more common encapsulated organisms becoming standard practice in asplenic individuals.

The spleen protects against infection not only by performing a filtering function, but also by producing specific antibodies against the polysaccharide antigens which lead to opsonization and destruction in reticuloendothelial tissues. The filtering function is probably the more important in preventing overwhelming infection.

By far the most clinically significant organism is *Streptococcus pneumoniae*. More than 50% of the major infections are caused by this organism. Although it is commonly thought that the highest risk of OPSI is within 2 years of splenectomy, this is a misconception. The risk is lifelong, with many of the infections occurring between 10 and 30 years after splenectomy, and the most commonly affected age group is 30–49. Therefore, signs of infection in asplenic patients should be treated as a serious medical emergency. Urgent administration of broad-spectrum antibiotics should follow the drawing of blood samples for culture.

## Prophylaxis after Splenectomy

Recommendations for prophylaxis, based on UK guidelines last updated in 2002, are summarized in Table 10.3. In general terms, no large trials prove the efficacy of the immunizations; however, strong evidence supports a role for such immunization in children undergoing splenectomy for sickle cell disease with a significant reduction in pneumococcal sepsis after vaccination. In adult populations, although breakthrough infections do occur, most episodes of OPSI occur in non-immunized or immunosuppressed patients.

Immunization with polyvalent pneumococcal vaccine and Haemophilus B and Meningococcal C vaccine should occur 2 weeks before elective splenectomy or, if not possible, as soon as feasible, at least 2 weeks post splenectomy. Influenza vaccine should be administered yearly. The UK guidelines recommend lifelong penicillin prophylaxis for asplenic patients. Prophylactic penicillin has been observed to decrease OPSI from S. pneumoniae in patients who have undergone splenectomy for Hodgkin's disease. There is little evidence that this is effective on a population basis, as breakthrough infections and resistance have been reported.

TABLE 10.3. Recommendations for immunization.

| Vaccine | Revaccination |
|---|---|
| Pneumococcal polyvalent vaccine | 5 years |
| Hemophilus influenza B conjugate | Unknown |
| Meningococcal C conjugate | Unknown |
| Influenza | Yearly |

Current evidence suggests that this guideline has not been implemented widely, and, even when attempted, compliance is generally poor. Guidelines from other organizations or countries suggest administration of penicillin for the first 2–5 years, but given that more infections occur after this period, this recommendation is hard to support. Many pediatricians support penicillin prophylaxis for 3–5 years after splenectomy in children.

What is clear is that suspected infections should be treated rapidly and aggressively, and asplenic patients should be given a supply of antibiotics to self-administer, particularly if traveling. Dog and other animal bites should be treated with a 5-day course of amoxicillin and clavulanic acid (or erythromycin in allergic patients) to protect against Capnocytophaga canimorsus. Malaria prophylaxis is essential when traveling to endemic areas due to the far greater incidence of aggressive malarial infection (and other infestations such as babesiosis) with a higher morbidity and mortality in asplenic individuals.

## Splenic Autotransplantation

As indicated above, the spleen is important for the removal of polysaccharide-encapsulated bacteria. There is conflicting evidence as to whether autotransplantation of splenic tissue, mainly in the trauma patient, helps to reduce OPSI. Certainly, there is no evidence that autotransplantation is harmful.

Studies indicate a better antibody response to pneumococcal vaccine in splenectomized patients who have undergone autotransplantation. Autotransplantation does not restore the splenic clearance function, which may be a consequence of a much lower blood flow through transplanted tissue than through the normal spleen. The enhanced antibody response may allow better opsonization of capsular polysaccharides and clearance by mononuclear cells elsewhere. In the clearance hierarchy, partial splenectomy or splenorrhaphy are superior to autotransplantation, which in turn is superior to an absence of splenic tissue.

The favored site of autotransplantation is an omental pouch, and the larger the ultimate volume of splenic tissue, the better the immunological function. Complications are rare although focal abscess formation has been described.

Splenic autotransplantation is therefore recommended in the trauma patient. Most experimental work has shown that maintenance of the tissue structure of the autotransplant is crucial, because splenosis after splenic trauma secondary to spillage and growth of splenocytes does not confer this immunologic protection. The splenic tissue should be placed in omental pouches and a significant volume of the spleen should be transplanted.

There are clear immunologic benefits associated with partial splenectomy. A minimum of approximately 25% of splenic weight with a good blood supply is required to maintain splenic immune function.

## Selected Readings

Clavien PA, Sarr MG, Fong U (2008) Atlas of upper gastrointestinal and hepato-pancreato-biliary surgery. Springer-Verlag Berlin and Heidelberg: (in press)

Davies JM, Barnes R, Milligan D, et al. (2002) Update of guidelines for the prevention and treatment of infection in patients with an absent or dysfunction spleen. Clin Med 2:440–443

Katz SC, Pachter HL (2006) Indications for splenectomy. Am Surg 72:565–580

Moore EE, Cogbill TH, Jurkovich GH, et al. (1995) Organ injury scaling: spleen and liver. J Trauma 38:323–324

Leonard AS, Giebink GS, Baesl TJ, et al. (1980) The overwhelming post-splenectomy sepsis problem. World J Surg 4:423–432

# 11
# Cyst and Abscess of the Spleen

**Luis Poggi and Juan Luis Calisto**

## Pearls and Pitfalls

- Most splenic cysts are benign; true primary or metastatic cystic lesions in the spleen are rare.
- Splenomegaly is usually seen with cysts larger than 6 cm.
- Symptomatic splenic cysts or those larger than 5 cm should be treated by operative intervention.
- An increased serum level of Ca 19.9 in a patient with a cystic lesion of the spleen suggests an epithelial cyst.
- Immunization is required in all patients in whom a splenectomy is planned.
- Laparoscopic approach should be attempted in most/all patients and converted to the open approach if necessary.
- Operative treatment can involve partial splenectomy trying to preserve the spleen, or total splenectomy if necessary.

## *Splenic abscess*

- Of infectious origin in the vast majority.
- Endocarditis and intravenous drug abuse should be thought of in a patient with a splenic abscess, especially if there are multiple abscesses.

K.I. Bland et al. (eds.), *Surgery of the Pancreas and Spleen*, DOI: 10.1007/978-1-84996-369-5_11,
© Springer-Verlag London Limited 2011

- Computed tomography is recommended, because its sensitivity is 95%; ultrasonography is less sensitive (75–90%).
- Small splenic abscesses maybe treated non-operatively with antibiotics; if no improvement occurs, interventional therapy (splenectomy or percutaneous drainage) is needed.
- Percutaneous drainage should be used only in selected patients (high risk, poor general status, malnutrition) due to its high recurrence rate.
- The risk of overwhelming postsplenectomy sepsis (OPS) is greater in children and in the immunosuppressed. Prophylaxis should be directed at the encapsulated bacteria (meningococcus, H. influenza, and pneumococcus).

# Introduction

Splenic cysts are usually asymptomatic, while abscesses always have an infectious cause and symptoms are first related to the underlying disease rather than the abscess itself. Splenic cysts are not the most common splenic pathology, because hematologic splenic pathology is by far more frequent.

# Splenic Cysts

Splenic cysts are an uncommon disease; there are few reports in literature, and most are anecdotal. Splenic cysts are generally asymptomatic, but some patients present with left upper quadrant pain related usually to the mass effect and local pressure created on other adjacent organs.

The first step in approaching what appears to be a splenic cyst is usually to determine whether the cystic lesion is a primary cyst or a pseudocyst. Primary splenic cysts have an epithelial lining, while pseudocysts lack an epithelial lining and are contained within a connective tissue capsule. Often, however, the diagnosis cannot be made preoperatively but only suspected.

# Splenic Abscess

The first description of splenic abscess comes from Hippocrates. Grand-Moursel made the first detailed description of the disease with a case series of 57 patients published in 1885. Due to its role in the circulatory system, the spleen is exposed to many infectious agents. Infectious processes are usually the cause of an abscess in the spleen. The most frequent etiologies of splenic abscess are endocarditis and intravenous drug abuse; immunosuppressed patients are affected more commonly by this condition. A splenic abscess can be caused by bacteria or fungi or they can be aseptic.

Symptoms of splenic abscess frequently involve spiking fever and pain in the left upper quadrant radiating to the back, but on occasion, the patient may have no pain. Splenic abscess is a disease that can be difficult to diagnose and requires a high index of suspicion. Splenic abscess can occur after traumatic subcapsular hematomas, infection of a parasitic cyst, or most commonly by hematologic dissemination due to sepsis.

The more common reported infectious agents include *E. coli*, *Klebsiella pneumoniae*, *Enterococcus spp.*, *Streptococcus viridans*, and *Staphylococcus aureus*, but *Pseudomona spp.*, *Brucella melitensis*, *TBC*, *Salmonella*, *Actinomyces*, and even superinfection of necrotic malignant splenic neoplasms have been reported. Culture of the purulent fluid is crucial to determine the appropriate antibiotic; it is recommended to take samples even if the collection does not seem to be a frank, purulent abscess. Hydatid disease of the spleen, though uncommon, still occurs, and superimposed infection of a hydatid cyst can develop. One must also remember that splenic abscesses are often accompanied by concomitant hepatic abscesses, especially if the etiology involves a hematologic infectious etiology.

## *Classification of Splenic Cysts*

Splenic cysts are rare, and most are benign. They are best divided in parasitic and nonparasitic cysts (Table 11.1).

TABLE 11.1. Classification.

**Abscess classification**

Pyogenic and bacterial

Infected parasitic

Infected hematoma

Mycotic

**Morgenstern's cyst classification**

(A) Parasitic

    Hydatid

Cysticercosis

(B) Nonparasitic

Congenital[a]

| | |
|---|---|
| | Mesothelial |
| | Transitional |
| Neoplastic | Epidermoid epithelium |
| | Endothelial origin |
| | • Lymphangioma |
| | • Hemangioma |
| | Primary cysts |
| | Metastasis with cystic degeneration |
| Traumatic | Lymphomas |
| Degenerative | Related to subcapsular hematomas |
| | Post infarction cysts |

[a]Those with a trabeculated lining despite histology.

Nonparasitic cysts can be divided further into benign and malignant cysts. The classification of parasitic cysts is non-problematic, but classification of the non parasitic cysts introduces some difficulties. Martin's classification is simple and is based on the presence (or absence) of an epithelial lining; however, the problem with this classification is that a misdiagnosis can be made if a careful detailed search for the presence of a lining is not made. Distinguishing between the different types of cysts is not always possible, and the crucial differentiation from a pseudocyst cannot always be made with assurance. Intracystic pressure can also distort the histology and may lead to a pressure necrosis of the epithelium, leaving some or much of the cyst wall denuded of its epithelial lining. Fowler's classification includes non parasitic cysts as neoplasms (although many are not really neoplasms); this classification also states that the absence of the lining qualifies many cysts as secondary and are classified as traumatic cysts or pseudocysts.

Recently, Morgenstern has addressed non parasitic cysts; he suggests that cysts with epithelial, transitional, or mesothelial histology are congenital in origin, and if histology is not conclusive or available, a trabeculated, fluid-filled cyst should be classified as a congenital cyst. We believe this classification is useful and recommend its use.

*Parasitic splenic cysts:* Parasitic cysts of the spleen are very rare except in endemic zones. The more common parasitic splenic cysts are the hydatid or echinococcal cysts and less frequently cysticercosis. To diagnose hydatid cysts, the Western Blot technique looking for specific parasitic proteins has a sensitivity that approaches 100%. When combined with imaging modalities that suggest a parasitic cyst, such as a thick wall with a complex cystic mass containing multiple septae and daughter cysts characteristic of hydatid cysts, one can make a firm diagnosis. On imaging and at operation, cystic content is usually liquid and contains visible parasitic membranes; in addition, calcification or semisolid components may be seen, depending on its chronicity.

*Non parasitic splenic cysts*: We classify congenital cysts as those with an epithelial lining (remember, it might be discontinuous with areas of no discernible epithelial lining) and those that have a characteristic white, trabeculated interior.

In contrast, hemangiomas, lymphangiomas, primary neo-plasms, or cystic metastases represent the neoplastic splenic cysts. Traumatic splenic cysts represent another type of splenic cyst and follow a known or presumed traumatic injury to the spleen; the cyst usually begins as a subcapsular hema-toma that resolves eventually but leaves a pseudocystic cav-ity; these traumatic splenic cysts have no epithelial lining and are really "pseudo" cysts.

Splenic infarcts can undergo cystic transformation and lead to a splenic "pseudo" cyst. While tumor biomarkers are usually not indicated at the time of initial evaluation, an increase in serum CA19-9 suggests the presence of an epithe-lial cyst. For complex, multi-loculated cystic masses, exclusion of a parasitic origin by serum markers is prudent.

## Classification of Splenic Abscess

Bryant proposes an etiologic classification for splenic abscesses based on five categories: (1) hematogenous origin as with endocarditis or intravenous drug abuse; (2) contiguous spread of infection from an adjacent source; (3) hemoglobinopathies, as in sickle cell anemia disease; (4) immunodeficiencies as in AIDS; and (5) abdominal trauma. Splenic abscesses can be subclassified into bacterial, mycotic, or parasitic.

# Clinical Presentation of Cystic Splenic Lesions

Diagnosis of a cystic lesion of the spleen relies on a compre-hensive medical history, because physical findings are usually vague and non-specific. Emphasis should focus on recent travel history, place of birth and/or country in which the patient lives or has lived, nutritional/immunologic status, underlying diseases (especially hematologic disorders), and social habits (AIDS, intravenous drug abuse, alcoholism, etc.). The clinical presentation is often asymptomatic or relatively subclinical. Much, however, can be learned from a directed history. Fever and chills suggest an infectious etiology, especially in the immunosuppressed or HIV patient, while primarily systemic symptoms, such as weight loss, fatigue, and anorexia, are more suggestive of a neoplastic etiology. Presence of left upper quadrant pain is often related to the size of the cystic lesion and the rate of growth.

Physical examination, aside from the associated comorbidities, offers little specific help unless there is left upper quadrant tenderness and/or splenomegaly. Laboratory evaluation may show leukocytosis, but other suggestive findings are lacking. Tumor markers and parasitic serologies are not cost-effective in the initial laboratory evaluation unless the imaging suggests a neoplastic or parasitic etiology.

# Diagnosis

First, clinical suspicion must be high, because in the absence of left upper quadrant pain, few other symptoms point to the spleen. Chest radiographs may show a left pleural effusion or an elevated left hemidiaphragm in patients with splenic abscesses, but these remain indirect signs. The best diagnostic measures involve the imaging modalities of ultrasonography, CT, or MRI. Sensitivities of defining a cystic lesion as an abscess range from 75% to 95%. Primary pancreatic cysts usually appear as a unilocular, fluid-filled cyst, while post-traumatic splenic pseudocysts often have septae and a nonhomogeneous intracystic content. In contrast, the characteristic features of splenic abscess are an enhancing wall and/or local surrounding inflammation; often the intracystic components are non-homogeneous.

## *Treatment*

Treatment of most symptomatic splenic cystic lesions or cystic neoplasms usually involves a splenectomy, currently performed laparoscopically whenever possible. After splenectomy, patients should receive appropriate immunization against the encapsulated bacteria: pneumococcus species, hemophilus influenza, and meningococcus. This triple immunization is especially important in children, patients with hematologic disorders, and the immunosuppressed.

## Parasitic/Hydatid Splenic Cysts

Although splenectomy remains the definitive procedure of choice for hydatid disease of the spleen, a course of preoperative administration of anti-parasitic agents seems prudent. Then, during the splenectomy, great care should be taken to avoid intraoperative spillage of intracystic contents because of the possibility of an anaphylactic response or local parasitic dissemination. Attempts at a splenic-preserving resection do not seem warranted for this disorder, especially with the potential for intraoperative spillage of cystic contents. While an initial attempt at a laparoscopic splenectomy seems warranted, the surgeon should have a low threshold for conversion to an open procedure if spillage of intracystic contents cannot be assured by a fully laparoscopic approach.

## Traumatic Splenic Pseudocysts and Simple Epithelial Cysts

When limited to one pole of the spleen, an attempt at a partial splenectomy, if technically feasible, seems warranted, especially in children, provided the entire cyst and its epithelial lining can be removed. Unroofing of these cysts with only peritoneal marsupialization have a definite incidence of recurrence, and thus, most experts suggest complete resection of the cyst.

## Splenic Abscess

Treatment of splenic abscess is more controversial. For most patients, splenectomy seems most prudent, especially when there are multiple abscesses. In contrast, when the abscess is small or there are miliary abscesses, a trial of intravenous anti-biotics is reasonable; if no improvement occurs, splenectomy can be performed. Management of the immunocompromised patient with a single fungal abscess or the critically ill patient, percutaneous image-guided drainage, culture of cystic con-tents, and focused anti-fungal or antibiotic therapy remains an option to operative splenectomy; however, recurrence or inability to eradicate the abscess is a distinct possibility and may necessitate later splenectomy. One must also remember to treat the primary source of sepsis causing the abscess as well.

## Our Experience

Over the last 21 years, we have managed 19 patients with cystic disorders of the spleen (Table 11.2). Three young patients had epithelial cysts with pain and an abdominal mass. CT showed cystic lesions of 13–25 cm in diameter (Fig. 11.1a); all underwent successful laparoscopic resection. Pathologic examination showed a trabeculated lining of the cyst wall (Fig. 11.1b). Two were hydatid cysts in patients from

TABLE 11.2. Institutional experience with cystic lesions of the spleen.

| | |
|---|---|
| **Splenic abscesses** | **8 patients** |
| Infected hydatid cyst | 4 |
| Infected hematoma | 4 |
| **Splenic cysts** | **11 patients** |
| Epithelial cysts | 3 |
| Hydatid cysts | 2 |
| Post traumatic pseudocysts | 2 |
| Post infarction cyst | 1 |
| Cystic endometrioma | 1 |
| Cystic lymphoma | 1 |
| Multiple cystic lymphangiomas | 1 |

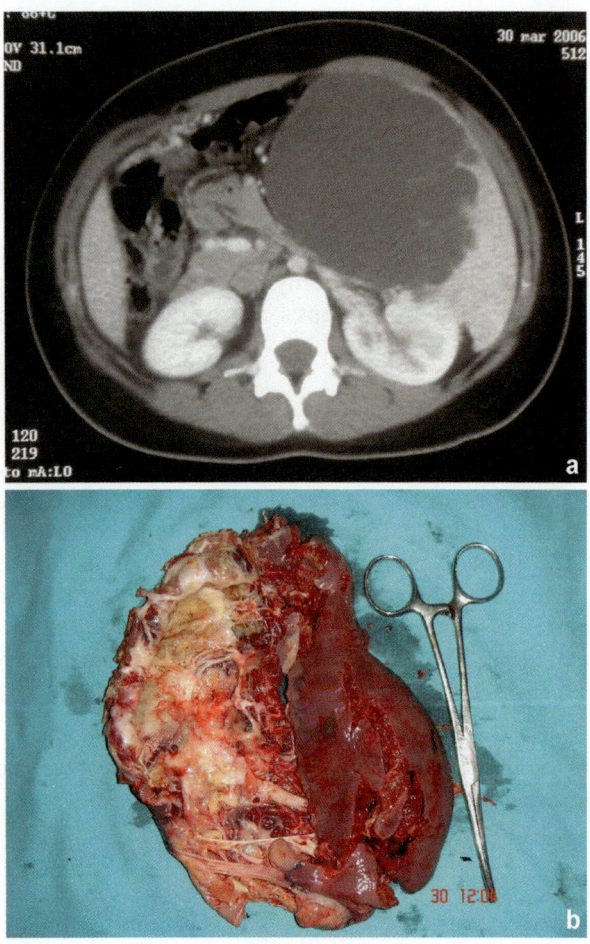

FIGURE 11.1. Epithelial cyst. (**a**) CT appearance. (**b**) Gross pathologic specimen.

the cattle zones (Fig. 11.2). Two patients proved to have splenic pseudocysts after a history of left upper quadrant trauma, while another had a previous splenic infarction that liquefied; these patients all had trabeculated cystic areas of resolving hematoma. The last three had cystic neoplasms,

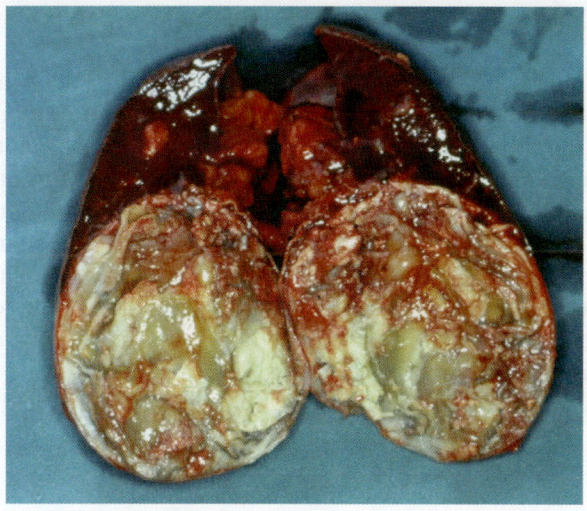

FIGURE 11.2. Splenic hydatid cyst.

including an endometrioma, a lymphoma, and one patient with multiple lymphangiomas.

## Complications of Splenectomy

Postoperative complications related to the operation and splenectomy include left-sided pleural effusion, subphrenic abscess, pancreatic fistula secondary to injury of the tail of the pancreas, and rarely a gastric leak secondary to devascularization/stomach injury at the site of the short gastric vessels. Specific problems related to removing the spleen involve thrombocytosis and overwhelming postsplenectomy sepsis (OPSS).

### Thrombocytosis

The platelet count increases in all patients after splenectomy. Most experts do not treat this thrombo-cytosis until the platelet count reaches one million; then treatment with anti-platelet agents seems warranted.

## OPSS

Although rare, OPSS can be aggressive and rapidly fatal. OPSS may start as a non-specific, flu-like prodrome but progress rapidly to bacteremic septic shock, acute renal failure, and disseminated intravascular coagulation. This syndrome is more likely to occur in children but can also involve adults, especially if immunosuppressed. Any febrile illness in a patient after a previous splenectomy should be treated aggressively. Patients and their families who have undergone splenectomy should be warned about this possibility and counseled in its recognition.

## Selected Readings

Chang KC, Chuah SK, Changchien CS (2006) Clinical characteristics and prognostic factors of splenic abscess: a review of 67 cases in a single medical center of Taiwan. World J Gastroenterol 12:460–464

Fowler RH (1953) Nonparasitic benign cystic tumors of the spleen. Int Abst Surg 96:209–227

Green BT (2001) Splenic abscess: report of six cases and review of the literature. Am Surg 67:80–85

Hao M (2006) Management of splenic pseudocysts following trauma: a retrospective case series. Am J Surg 191:631–634.

Martin JW (1958) Congenital splenic cysts. Am J Surg 96:302–308

Morgenstern L (2002) Nonparasitic splenic cysts: pathogenesis, classification, and treatment. Am Coll Surg 194:306–314

Sánchez López JD, Cerquella Hernández C (1998) Quiste epitelial esplénicoy elevación sérica del Ca 19.9. Arch Cir Gen Dig 12:5

# Part IV
# Spleen—Malignant

# 12
# Malignant Diseases of the Spleen

**Patricio Burdiles and Yaira Lopez**

## Pearls and Pitfalls

- Malignant diseases affecting the spleen, especially primary splenic neoplasms, are extremely rare.
- Lymphomas and lymphoproliferative disorders are the most prevalent diseases involving the spleen, while hemangiosarcomas are the most prevalent primary neoplasms of the spleen.
- Hemangioma is the most frequent benign, primary neoplasm of the spleen.
- Splenic malignancies maybe asymptomatic and are usually found serendipitously during an image assessment for unrelated conditions.
- Local symptoms are painful splenomegaly, hypersplenism, or palpable mass.
- The presence of "B" symptoms (fever, night sweats, and weight loss) is clinically relevant.
- Splenectomy either through classic laparotomy or more recently using a laparoscopic approach is indicated in solid neoplasms affecting the spleen as long as there is no invasion to adjacent organs.
- If a laparoscopic approach is chosen and an intact specimen is important for pathologic analysis (e.g., Hodgkin's lymphoma), the extraction can be made through a small peri-umbilical or suprapubic incision.

K.I. Bland et al. (eds.), *Surgery of the Pancreas and Spleen*, DOI: 10.1007/978-1-84996-369-5_12, © Springer-Verlag London Limited 2011

- For most solid splenic masses, only the benign hemangioma with typical characteristics at magnetic resonance imaging (MRI) can be followed non-operatively with confidence.
- Metastatic neoplasms of the spleen are exceptionally rare and are generally secondary to advanced neoplasms, often ovarian.

# Epidemiology

Primary neoplasms affecting the spleen are extremely rare in any surgical practice compared with the more common hematologic diseases. Currently, in most reported series of elective splenectomy, malignant cases usually comprise fewer than 25% of the splenectomies and are usually for lymphomas and some leukemias. Malignancies of spleen are distributed similarly in both sexes and usually affect the fifth and sixth decades of life.

# Classification

The spleen is involved in the lymphoproliferative or myeloproliferative diseases but only rarely with primary benign neoplasms, malignant neoplasms, or metastatic spleen lesions. Table 12.1 shows a classification of malignant lesions of the spleen.

## Lymphoproliferative Diseases

Lymphomas affect the spleen in approximately 20–30% of patients as part of a more diffuse, systemic disease affecting lymph nodes and bone marrow. Hodgkin's disease is a highly curable lymphoma which differs from other lymphoproliferative diseases in its predictable, stepwise progression from one nodal group to another. Hodgkin's disease often presents

TABLE 12.1.   Malignant diseases of the spleen.

1. Lymphoproliferative diseases

    - Lymphoma (Hodgkin's, non-Hodgkin's, marginal zone lymphoma)

    - Chronic lymphocytic leukemia

    - Hairy cell leukemia

    - Plasmacytoma

    - Waldenström's macroglobulinemia

2. Myeloproliferative diseases

    - Chronic myelogenous leukemia

    - Myelofibrosis (agnogenic myeloid metaplasia)

    - Polycythemia vera Primary neoplasms

3. Primary neoplasms

    - Sarcomas (hemangiosarcoma, lymphosarcoma, fibrosarcoma, leiomyosarcoma, Kaposi's sarcoma)

    - Plasmacytoma

    - Malignant fibrous histiocytoma

4. Metastatic neoplasms

    - Ovary

    - Breast

    - Lung

    - Melanoma

above the diaphragm with typical enlarged and firm lymph nodes affecting the neck and mediastinum and limited to lymph nodal involvement in 85% of patients. When the disease occurs below the diaphragm, the spleen is the first organ to be affected and subsequently other lymph nodal groups. It is estimated that 35% of patients with stage I or stage II

Hodgkin's disease have occult splenic involvement. While in the past splenectomy was part of the staging laparotomy for Hodgkin's disease, currently it is indicated only rarely because of more effective chemotherapy.

Primary splenic lymphomas are extremely rare (<1% of patients with lymphoma). Non-Hodgkin's lymphomas are more frequent causes of splenic involvement than Hodgkin's lymphomas and are predominantly B-cell lymphomas that present usually with lymph node enlargement and rarely with fever, night sweats, and weight loss.

A special type of lymphoma called marginal zone lymphoma is a unique neoplasm comprising 1–2% of all non-Hodgkin's lymphomas and up to 20% of lymphoproliferative disorders diagnosed after splenectomy. This B-cell lymphoma is considered a low-grade malignancy because of its indolent clinical course and relatively good long-term prognosis with a 5-year survival of 65%. Marginal zone lymphoma is characterized by splenomegaly, bone marrow involvement, and circulating lymphocytes with an irregular cytoplasmic border distinct from hairy cell leukemia; this lymphoma appears to arise from different subsets of splenic marginal zone B cells.

Chronic lymphocytic leukemia (CLL) is another lymphoproliferative disease that can affect the spleen. Many of these patients live for years with no treatment; some patients develop quite impressive splenomegaly with hypersplenism. Although splenectomy in this condition is not always rewarded by improvement in the pancytopenia, thrombocytopenia may respond in half of patients. Splenectomy is usually offered more for symptomatic relief of this large abdominal mass.

In this group is also hairy cell leukemia, a chronic B-cell disease presenting with pancytopenia and splenomegaly. Neoplastic cells with hair-like projections are evident in the peripheral blood and bone marrow. Medical treatment with chlorodeoxyadenosine has changed prognosis markedly by inducing a complete remission in 85% of patients. Splenectomy should be considered only in patients with painful splenomegaly.

## Myeloproliferative Diseases

Chronic myelogenous leukemia (CML) accounts for 30% of all leukemias in adults. Splenomegaly is present in 50–75% of these patients. The degree of splenomegaly correlates with total body white blood cell mass and blood granulocyte count. Complications of the splenomegaly include splenic infarction or rupture, hypersplenism, and, most commonly, painful splenomegaly. Splenectomy can help to improve quality of life when these complications appear but has an appreciable morbidity and mortality and does not delay the onset of blastic transformation or prolong survival.

Myelofibrosis (agnogenic myeloid metaplasia [AMM]) is another rare condition affecting pre-dominantly men in the seventh decade. AMM is characterized by splenomegaly, leukoerythroblastic transformation and poikilocytosis in the peripheral blood, and hypocellularity in the bone marrow. Primary AMM has a 5-year survival of 60%. Secondary AMM is the consequence of a transformation of polycythemia rubra vera or essential thrombocythemia to this myelofibrotic state with survival for this disorder being <2 years. Splenectomy is reserved for when splenomegaly impairs quality of life, because postoperative morbidity and mortality is high (about 20%) secondary to bleeding, thrombosis, and sepsis.

## Primary Malignancies of the Spleen

These groups of neoplasms are exceptionally rare, and only a few hundred cases have been reported in the literature.

Hemangiosarcoma, the most frequent primary splenic malignancy, presents with anemia, left upper abdominal pain, and splenomegaly. At the time of diagnosis, many patients already have metastases to the liver, lung, and bones. This aggressive neoplasm has a peculiar tendency to bleed because of spontaneous rupture of the spleen. The prognosis is dismal with 80% of patients dead before the first year and with essentially no survival at 5 years. When suspected, splenectomy and aggressive chemo-radiotherapy are indicated. Other primary malignancies of the spleen include lymphangiosarcomas, liposarcomas, and hemangiopericytoma, but they are even rarer, and only anecdotal cases have been reported.

Important in the differential diagnosis are benign tumors of the spleen which present a diagnostic challenge and dilemma that can often be resolved only by splenectomy. Splenic hemangioma, although rare, is the most common benign primary neoplasm of the spleen. These neoplasms are always asymptomatic and discovered serendipitously. As with liver hemangiomas, splenic hemangiomas are small and cavernous; they appear to originate from the red pulp and become symptomatic only if they are large (sometimes with hypersplenism or portal hypertension), compress adjacent structures, or rupture. In such patients, splenectomy is indicated; otherwise, if the splenic imaging is characteristic, observational therapy alone is indicated.

Other benign vascular disorders of the spleen include peliosis, a rare condition occurring mostly in men (75%) with debilitating illnesses such as tuberculosis or cancer. Multiple, small, blood-filled cysts are visible throughout the entire spleen which is usually of a normal size. Some of these patients die because of sudden splenic rupture and consequently lethal hemorrhage. Splenectomy is recommended when peliosis is found at laparotomy. Another rare vascular neoplasm is lymphangioma, a subcapsular lesion which can involve the entire organ and cause hypersplenism and/or symptomatic painful splenomegaly. Hamartomas are embryonic in their origin and are considered to be a non-neoplastic disorder. Although usually asymptomatic, they can sometimes become clinically relevant when splenomegaly, a palpable abdominal mass, or hypersplenism is present.

## Metastatic Neoplasms of the Spleen

Splenic metastases are present in up to 7% of autopsies in patients with advanced cancer. Splenic involvement is almost always associated with extensive metastatic disease, including the peritoneal surface, lung, liver, and bone marrow. Melanoma, breast, ovarian, lung, and colorectal cancer are the most frequent neoplasms that affect the spleen by metastatic hematogenous spread. Solitary splenic metastases are extremely rare, but when present, more than half of the neoplasms are gynecologic in origin. Careful assessment for metastases is necessary before splenectomy is entertained.

## Clinical Presentation

The classic symptoms related to lymphomas include fever, nocturnal sweating, generalized weakness (called B symptoms), weight loss, and painful tenderness affecting the upper left quadrant of the abdomen associated with splenomegaly. Benign and malignant neoplasms are usually asymptomatic and maybe found as an unexpected mass on abdominal imaging for another disorder. Rarely, they may present as symptomatic, painful splenomegaly or a palpable mass in the left upper abdominal quadrant. More malignant neoplasms tend to present in older patients than do benign neoplasms. Malignant splenic neoplasms are larger in size and often associated with coagulation disorders, anemia, and thrombocytopenia, which complicate the splenectomy. Hemangiosarcoma and other disorders carry the risk of splenic rupture and clinically significant hemorrhage.

## Diagnosis

The mainstay of diagnosis involves cross-sectional imaging combined with hematologic investigation. Abdominal ultrasonography or computed tomography (CT) usually shows a hypoechoic mass involving the spleen. In conjunction with the clinical evaluation and a thorough physical examination, further CT assessment of thorax, abdomen, and pelvis is indicated in order to establish the stage of the disease.

In the differential diagnosis, hemangioma of the spleen should be excluded because hemangioma requires no intervention. The classic image of splenic hemangioma on magnetic resonance (MR) shows a heterogeneous mass of high signal intensity due to its content of water at T2 MR image, with a slow, centripetal pattern of peripheral enhancement and central hypointense radial lines due to fibrosis at T1 MR image. This appearance is pathognomonic and is the only disorder that allows conservative management as long as the patient remains asymptomatic.

## Patient Management

The practice of splenectomy as part of the staging process in lymphomas has decreased markedly, because imaging assessment is currently very accurate and reliable enough to permit an appropriate decision process. The usual indications for splenectomy are hypersplenism-associated cytopenias, relief of symptoms due to massive splenomegaly, or rarely as a salvage procedure when chemotherapy has failed. This strategy is accepted and used in the management of lymphoproliferative disorders.

Unfortunately, splenectomy represents the only method to obtain an accurate histologic diagnosis of a solitary solid mass affecting the spleen. Open splenectomy allows an optimal analysis of the whole organ by the pathologist. In contrast, laparoscopic splenectomy is attractive because of its minimally invasive approach, but this approach usually requires fragmentation (morcellation) of the splenic tissue inside the extraction bag to avoid a laparotomy for taking out the resected specimen; a relatively small supra-pubic incision can be used to extract the bag with an intact spleen such as in the case of Hodgkin's disease. It is important to avoid rupture of the spleen or spillage of any fragment of splenic tissue into the peritoneal cavity which could result in splenosis or recurrent disease. The outcomes of splenectomy for myeloproliferative disorders are poor; postoperative morbidity is about 50% (mostly respiratory and bleeding) and postoperative mortality approaches 15–20%. When a laparoscopic approach is possible, morbidity is decreased. Laparoscopic splenectomy is contraindicated usually for large splenomegaly >20 cm, because of the difficulties in accessing the hilum, mobilization of ligaments, and managing retrieval of the spleen.

As with all splenectomies, consideration of bacterial vaccines is highly recommended in an attempt to prevent post-splenectomy sepsis, especially in the immunocompromised host.

## Selected Readings

Berge T (1974) Splenic metastases: frequencies and patterns. Acta Path Microbiol Scand 82:499–506

Burch M, Misra M, Phillips EH (2005) Splenic malignancy: a minimally invasive approach. Cancer J 11:36–42

Coon WW (1998) Surgical aspects of splenic disease and lymphoma. Curr Probl Surg 35:547–632

Friedman RL, Hiatt JR, Korman JL, et al. (1997) Laparoscopic or open splenectomy for hematologic disease: which approach is superior? J Am Coll Surg 185:49–54

Oscier D, Owen R, Johnson S (2005) Splenic marginal zone lymphoma. Blood Rev 19:39–51

Wick MR, Smith SL, Scheicthauer BW, et al. (1982) Primary nonlymphoreticular malignant neoplasms of the spleen. Am J Surg Pathol 6:229–242

# Part V
# Minimally Invasive Procedures

# 13
# Advanced Gastric and Pancreatic Laparoscopic Procedures

**Pedro Ferraina, Luis A. Durand, Ariel Ferraro, Miguel Caracoche, and Mario S. Nahmod**

## Pearls and Pitfalls

Laparoscopic gastric surgery

- Laparoscopic resection of gastric pathology is common in some Asian countries, but laparoscopic surgery for gastric cancer has not yet achieved worldwide acceptance.
- Preliminary results suggest that in expert hands, this approach is safe, technically feasible, and achieves results comparable to that for open gastric resection with a shortened hospitalization.
- The specific advantages for laparoscopic access are a minimal access approach, less postoperative pain, better recovery, and less morbidity.
- Laparoscopic resection is well-accepted for gastrointestinal stromal neoplasms, but less so for formal gastrectomies because of lack of appropriate candidates and lack of experience.
- Early gastric cancer (limited to the mucosal and submucosal spread) is suited ideally for a laparoscopic or laparoendoscopic approach.
- Perforated or obstructing duodenal ulcers are ideal candidates for a laparoscopic approach.

K.I. Bland et al. (eds.), *Surgery of the Pancreas and Spleen*, DOI: 10.1007/978-1-84996-369-5_13, © Springer-Verlag London Limited 2011

Laparoscopic pancreatic surgery

- Laparoscopic staging of pancreatic cancer may show liver, peritoneal, or distant nodal disease precluding a curative resection thereby avoiding a laparotomy.
- In experienced hands, operative palliation of biliary obstruction by cholecystojejunostomy and future duodenal obstruction by gastroenterostomy can be performed laparoscopically.
- Laparoscopic distal pancreatectomy has been performed with good results for benign disorders or selected pancreatic neoplasms, especially cystic neoplasms or neuroendocrine neoplasms.
- Laparoscopic approaches to enucleation of insulinomas are ideal.
- Although laparoscopic and laparoendoscopic approaches have been described for transgastric drainage of pancreatic pseudocysts, they offer little advantage to endoscopic internal drainage.
- Selected patients with established infected necrosis or non-resolving sterile necrosis can be managed by minimal access techniques of necrosectomy.

# Laparoscopic Gastric Surgery

Laparoscopic gastric resection was first reported for a chronic gastric ulcer in 1992 and was soon followed by laparoscopic gastrectomy for cancer in 1993. Since then, laparoscopic techniques have been used in an ever-increasing variety of gastric resective procedures, including primarily benign gastric lesions but, in some centers, in early gastric cancer and advanced cancer as well. These laparoscopic approaches include totally laparoscopic, laparoscopic-assisted, and combined laparoscopic and endoluminal procedures.

The most common benign gastric neoplasms for which a laparoscopic approach is well accepted include gastrointestinal stromal tumors (GIST) and carcinoid neoplasms. However, other gastric lesions that may require excision are leiomyomas, large polyps, and pancreatic rests which can mimic a neoplasm. Gastric stromal neoplasms are most often present with mucosal ulceration that leads to gastrointestinal bleeding, but they may also be discovered incidentally during upper gastrointestinal endoscopy or cross-sectional imaging for some unrelated indication. The treatment is local excision with negative margins that can be accomplished with a wedge resection in most patients.

Most gastric GISTs are small and appropriate for laparoscopic removal. Laparoscopic excision of tumors >5 cm is somewhat controversial because of the increased likelihood of malignancy and potential difficulty with tumor manipulation. GISTs that occur in the distal antrum or prepyloric region may require antrectomy for removal unless they are based on a narrow stalk and are growing primarily extragastric. In contrast, the submucosal GISTs that extend primarily intraluminally are more difficult to locate and resect; despite their intraluminal location, they may still be based primarily on a narrow stalk or base, allowing wedge-type resection. Lesions arising at or near the gastroesophageal junction along the lesser curvature are often the most difficult to manage.

In addition to resection of gastric lesions, advanced techniques can also be applied to duodenal ulcer disease. While formal acid-reducing resections are uncommon today, perforated duodenal ulcers lend themselves well to a laparoscopic closure with or without a vascularized omental patching. Vagotomies, either truncal or proximal gastric vagotomy, can be performed simultaneously with relative ease in appropriately selected patients, often with either a pyloroplasty or loop gastroenterostomy, if needed. Similarly, an obstructing duodenal or pyloric channel ulcer can be treated by vagotomy and loop gastroenterostomy or pyloroplasty (if appropriate).

## *Laparoscopic Gastric Resection for Gastric Cancer*

Laparoscopic surgery for gastric cancer is more common in certain Asian countries, such as Japan and Korea because of both the higher incidence of this neoplasm in Asian countries and related screening practices which identify the disease at a much earlier state. Although laparoscopic surgery for gastric cancer has not yet achieved worldwide acceptance; it will soon follow.

Among patients with gastric cancer, those with early-stage cancers are the best candidates for laparoscopic surgery. Multiple types of laparoscopic and laparoendoscopic procedures for early gastric cancer have been developed. These procedures are categorized according to the extent of the lymph node dissection: laparoscopic local resection with or without lymph node dissection and laparoscopic gastrectomy with D1 or D2 lymph node dissection.

## Laparoscopic Local Resection for Gastric Cancer

There are two primary laparoscopic procedures for local resection of early gastric cancer: laparoscopic wedge resection and laparoendoscopic intragastric mucosal resection.

*Indications*: Laparoscopic local resection is used to treat early gastric cancer without lymph node metastasis in patients who are not candidates for endoscopic mucosal resection because of tumor size or location. Lymph node metastasis occurs in 2–5% of mucosal cancers and in up to 20% of submucosal cancers.

Laparoscopic wedge resection is used for cancers located on the anterior wall, lesser curvature, or greater curvature of the stomach. Laparoscopic intragastric mucosal resection is not performed frequently because of the technical difficulty of the procedure. However, it can be utilized to treat cancers on the posterior wall of the stomach or near the cardia or pylorus. For either approach, intraoperative endoscopic observation is required to localize the cancer and direct the resection.

*Laparoscopic wedge resection*: The technique for laparoscopic wedge resection of gastric lesions varies depending on the size of the lesion and its location. The lesion is elevated by grasping adjacent normal stomach. If the lesion is difficult to grasp or elevate, sutures placed in the gastric wall adjacent to the mass can be used for traction to facilitate placement of a stapler. An endoscopic linear cutting stapler is positioned under the lesion to obtain a sufficient margin of normal tissue. The gastric staple line can be inverted with interrupted or running absorbable suture. The resection specimen is placed in a bag and removed at the conclusion of the procedure. The specimen should be examined by the pathologist to ensure negative gross resection margins (Fig. 13.1). Post resection endoscopy will assume maintenance of an appropriate luminal size and lack of bleeding.

*Laparoendoscopic Intragastric Mucosal Resection*: Three balloon trocars are placed into the gastric lumen penetrating both the abdomen and stomach wall. The stomach then is insufflated with $CO_2$, and laparoscopic instruments are introduced. Mucosal resection is performed using forceps and electrocautery and/or laser under either laparoendoscopic or endoscopic observation. After resection, the specimen is extracted endoscopically, and each trocar site in the stomach is closed laparoscopically.

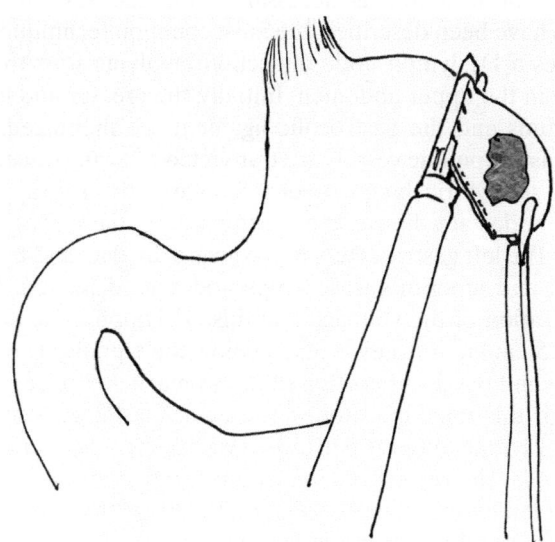

FIGURE 13.1. Laparoscopic wedge resection.

# Laparoscopic Gastrectomy for Gastric Cancer

*Indications:* Laparoscopic gastrectomy can be performed in three ways: totally laparoscopic, laparoscopic-assisted, and by a hand-assisted laparoscopic technique. The laparoscopic-assisted procedure is the most popular, because the resected specimen can be extracted from the abdominal cavity through a small laparotomy incision. These resections can be performed with perigastric lymph node dissection (D1) and extended lymph node dissection (D2).

Laparoscopic distal, proximal, and total gastrectomy are performed according to the location of the tumor and the depth of invasion as in open surgery. Compared with open surgery, laparoscopic gastrectomy offers several potential benefits, including less pain, less inflammatory response, faster recovery of gastrointestinal function, and a shorter hospital stay.

*Technique of laparoscopy-assisted distal gastrectomy:* To identify the oral margin of cancer, preoperative endoscopic clipping or tattooing is necessary. Although several techniques have been described, the most common technique also involves a D1 lymph node dissection involving four trocars placed in the upper abdomen. Initially, the greater and lesser omentums and the gastrocolic ligament are mobilized. The right gastroepiploic vessels are transected allowing dissection of the subpyloric lymph nodes. Similarly, the suprapyloric lymph nodes are dissected after transecting the right gastric artery. The left gastric artery and vein are divided, and the left cardiac and superior gastric lymph nodes are dissected. After mobilization of the stomach and this D1 lymph node dissection, a 5-cm laparotomy is made below the xiphoid. The duodenum and the distal portion of the stomach are exteriorized through this minilaparotomy. The actual distal gastrectomy with D1 lymph nodes is performed with a linear stapler extracorporally. The reconstruction by a Billroth-II method is also performed extracorporally (Fig. 13.2). This author prefers an extracorporeal anastomosis and performs an intracorporeal anastomosis only after a more distal gastrectomy, because a

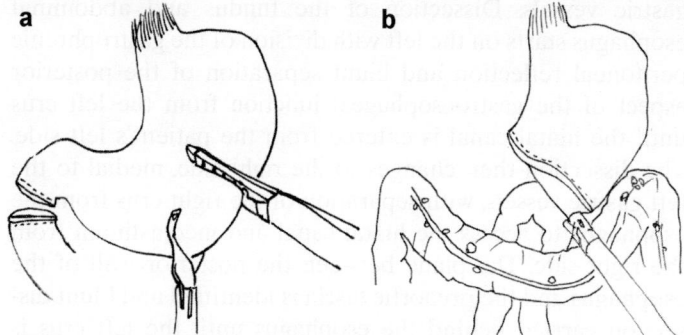

FIGURE 13.2. Proximal transection of the stomach. Gastrojejunostomy loop joined laparoscopically with GIA.

laparotomy is needed to remove the specimen. For markedly obese patients or those in whom the stomach and/or duodenum cannot be mobilized out of the wound, intracorporeal anastomosis can be performed using endoscopic stapling devices or a laparoscopic, hand-sewn technique.

*Laparoscopic Total D1 Gastrectomy:* Mobilization of the greater curvature involves detaching the entire greater omentum from the transverse colon or mesocolon. The crucial step facilitating this procedure involves downward traction on the transverse colon by a large atraumatic forceps. The mobilization proceeds from the right side (duodenum and hepatic flexure) to the inferior pole of the spleen and adjacent left paracolic gutter. This step is facilitated using a hand-assisted device, because a short laparotomy is required to remove the specimen. Thereafter, the short gastric vessels are transected with the harmonic dissector with preservation of the spleen, or if the tumor is located at the greater curvature, the spleen can be removed en bloc with the stomach, thereby avoiding the need to transect the short gastric vessels. On the right side, the right gastroepiploic vessels and the right gastric artery are transected similarly or clipped.

Next, the lesser omentum is divided, as close to the liver as possible, from the divided right gastric vessels up to the left gastric vessels. Dissection of the fundus and abdominal esophagus starts on the left with division of the gastrophrenic peritoneal reflection and blunt separation of the posterior aspect of the gastroesophageal junction from the left crus until the hiatal canal is entered from the patient's left side. The dissection then changes to the right side, medial to the left gastric vessels, with separation of the right crus from the esophagus to access the hiatal canal and mediastinum from the right side. The plane between the posterior wall of the esophagus and the preaortic fascia is identified and blunt dissection carried behind the esophagus until the left crus is reached, similar to the dissection for a laparoscopic Nissen fundoplication. At this stage, a sling passed around the mobilized esophagus is used to pull the esophagus away from the mediastinum to complete the posterior separation. Division of the posterior and anterior vagal trunks allows the surgeon to pull more of the mediastinal esophagus into the peritoneal cavity.

The next maneuver involves dissection of the celiac axis with division of the left gastric artery at its origin and division of the left gastric (coronary) vein. Identification of the celiac trunk requires retraction of the gastroesophageal junction inferiorly and to the left with inferior retraction of the superior margin of the pancreas. Dissection with a harmonic scalpel proceeds carefully until the origin of the left gastric artery is identified clearly. The left gastric artery and vein are clipped in continuity before the artery is divided (proximal to any lymph node mass), because insufficient space exists behind the artery to introduce the limb of the vascular stapler.

Next, the duodenum is transected with an endoscopic linear stapler after mobilization of the distal stomach as above; the specimen (and reconstruction) is then removed through an upper midline minilaparotomy or through the hand-assisted wound. A noncrushing clamp is placed across the esophagus approximately 2.5 cm proximal to the transection site. The esophagus is divided, and the specimen is removed through the wound.

Reconstruction, after total or subtotal gastrectomy for cancer, is performed best with a Roux-en-Y anastomosis. For reconstruction after total gastrectomy, a pursestring suture (2-0 polypropylene) is placed at the cut end of the esophagus, and the anvil of the circular stapler is introduced into the lumen of the esophagus, after which the pursestring is tied over the stem. We prefer a classic Hunt-Lawrence type pouch created from a Roux limb of the upper jejunum using an endoscopic stapler.

# Duodenal Ulcer Disease: Laparoscopic Treatment

*Perforated duodenal ulcer*: The current treatment for perforated duodenal ulcer in patients ≥40 years old involves closure of the perforation alone and acid suppression. In the younger patient, in whom the etiology is usually *Helicobacter pylori*, again treatment no longer involves gastrectomy and/ or vagotomy but rather control of the perforation and aggressive eradication of *H. pylori* infection. Laparoscopic closure of the perforation is ideally suited for this complication. Using three upper abdominal trocars, the perforation is almost always anterior and localized easily. One or two sutures placed laparoscopically will close the perforation easily. Next the abdomen is lavaged extensively both in the upper and lower regions to remove any extravasations. After this, a tongue of vascularized greater omentum can be swung up and fixed on top of the duodenal closure as reinforcement. If the perforation is >1 cm but <2 cm, a formal omental patch and/or plug can be considered. If the perforation is ≥2 cm, the procedure should probably be converted to an open exploration for classic repair; attempts at a laparoscopic gastrectomy or Roux limb patch may not be prudent for the very large perforations in these acutely ill patients because of the often added time needed.

Patients with bleeding duodenal ulcers requiring operative treatment are not good candidates for a laparoscopic approach because of difficulties with visualization of an actively bleeding vessel of this magnitude and the need for a precisely placed suture control.

## Laparoscopic Pancreatic Surgery

The first reports of the use of laparoscopy in pancreatic pathologies occurred in the 1980s and early 1990s directed at evaluation, biopsy, and staging of pancreatic malignancies. Subsequently, the technological improvements and experience have allowed a laparoscopic approach to resection of solid organs. At present, laparoscopic surgery of the pancreas is being investigated and developed actively in multiple centers around the world. While experience remains largely preliminary, the growing interest and experience primarily with distal pancreatectomy and enucleation of insulinomas shows that this approach offers the typical advances of a minimal access operation. Laparoscopic distal pancreatectomy will soon become the gold standard.

The present applications of a laparoscopic approach to pancreatic surgery include pathologies such as pancreatic cancer, neuroendocrine and cystic neoplasms, chronic pancreatitis, and complications of acute pancreatitis (Table 13.1). The advantages of the laparoscopic approach in explorations for many pancreatic diseases reside in the magnification of the visual field, a lesser systemic response to operation, and a shorter hospital stay. The disadvantage resides in the technical difficulty in carrying out pancreatic resections that require more advanced, technical skills.

The basic pancreatic exploration consists of the glandular exposure. The gastrocolic omentum is divided, preserving the gastroepiploic artery. The lesser sac is entered with exposure of the anterior wall of the pancreas, especially of the neck, body and tail of the gland. A special consideration in the approach of the tail of the pancreas is that the dissection should begin with the mobilization of the splenic flexure of the colon to respect the short gastric vessels (Fig. 13.3).

TABLE 13.1. Utility of the laparoscopic approach in the pancreatic pathologies.

| Pathology | Technique | |
| --- | --- | --- |
| Pancreatic cancer | Laparoscopic staging | |
| | Palliative procedures | Cholecystojejunostomy |
| | | Hepaticojejunostomy (loop or Roux limb) |
| | | Choledochoduodenostomy |
| | | Gastro-enterostomy |
| | Pancreaticoduodenectomy | |
| Cystic neoplasms | Pancreatic resection | Distal pancreatectomy with or without splenectomy |
| Insulinomas | Pancreatic resection | Insulinoma enucleation |
| Chronic pancreatitis | Pancreatic resection | Distal pancreatectomy with or without splenectomy |
| | Internal drainage of pancreatic pseudocyst | Pancreatic cyst-gastrostomy |
| | | Pancreatic cyst-jejunostomy |
| Acute pancreatitis | Necrosis debridement | Video-assisted necrosectomy |
| | Internal drainage of pancreatic pseudocyst | Pancreatic cyst-gastrostomy |
| | | Pancreatic cyst-jejunostomy |

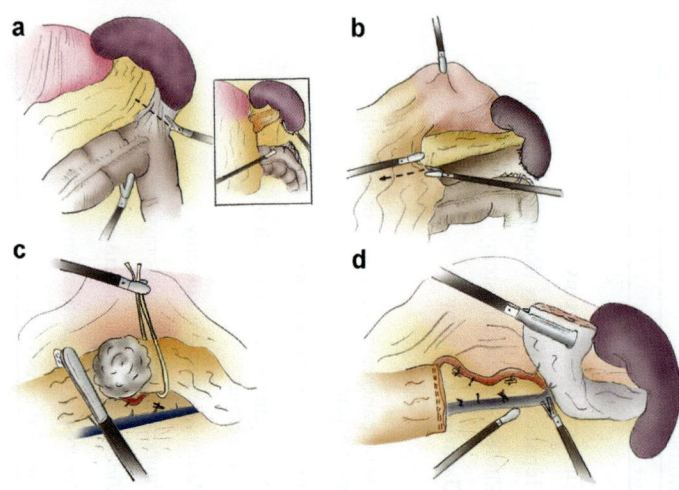

FIGURE 13.3. Laparoscopic distal pancreatectomy. (**a**) The splenic flexure of the colon is mobilized and the gastrocolic omentum divided. The splenocolic ligament must be mobilized for visualization of the pancreatic tail. (**b**) The inferior surface of the pancreas is dissected free and the spleen mobilized laterally, medially, and inferiorly. (**c**) The neck of the pancreas is transected with a linear stapler after the body and tail have been fully mobilized. (**d**) The spleen can be preserved by ligating all branches off the splenic artery and vein, or the spleen can be removed with the pancreas en bloc by ligating the splenic artery and vein proximally at the site of pancreatic parenchymal transection.

Correct preoperative staging is important for patients with pancreatic neoplasms and especially ductal cancer of the pancreas, because only 10% of patients will be candidates for resection with curative intent. Better methods of staging in combination with endoscopic techniques of internal biliary stenting to relieve the biliary obstruction will prevent unnecessary non-therapeutic laparotomies.

Because metastatic dissemination takes place primarily in liver, lymph nodes, and peritoneum, laparoscopic staging seems ideal for these neoplasms. The addition of laparoscopic ultrasonography allows further detection of intraparenchy-mal hepatic metastases and the evaluation of the local-regional extension of the tumor in the region of the portal and superior mesenteric veins. In addition, use of a laparoscopic approach to operative palliation (biliary bypass and gastroenterostomy) offers the patient palliation with less morbidity than obtained with open operative palliation.

Many pancreatic surgeons use a laparoscopic staging for patients with periampullary carcinomas with advanced local-regional extension without evidence of distant disease (T2-T3, Nx, Mo) and all presumably malignant neoplasms of the body and tail of the gland; use of staging laparoscopy in this latter group is especially important, because metastatic disease precluding a curative resection is found in at least 40% of patients with ductal cancer of the pancreas, and thereby obviating the need for open operative exploration. The patients with ampullary neoplasms or periampullary tumors < 2cm (T1, N0, M0) usually do not benefit by preoperative laparoscopic staging, because they usually will not have distant dissemination.

*Technique of laparoscopic staging*: The patient is placed supine with the legs spread and the surgeon positioned between the patient's legs. The access ports consist of three or four trocars; usually one or two 10 mm ports (umbilical, right subcostal) and two 5 mm ports (left subcostal and subiphoid). The entire abdominal cavity is inspected as well as the surface of the liver to determine the presence of peritoneal and hepatic metastasis. Laparoscopic ultrasonography can be used to look for intrahepatic metastases not evident by laparoscopic visualization alone. Subsequently, the pancreas can be exposed by entering the lesser sac through the gastrocolic ligament to expose the anterior wall of the pancreas. Laparoscopic ultrasonography will allow determination of the relationship between the pancreatic neoplasm and the extrahepatic portal venous system. In patients with locally advanced disease, laparoscopy-guided fine needle aspiration of the pancreatic lesion is usually done to confirm diagnosis, and then the corresponding palliative operation can be performed.

*Laparoscopic palliation of pancreatic cancer*: Using the same trocars as for staging and if possible, even proceeding at the time of laparoscopic staging, palliative procedures can be performed. Biliary bypass is accomplished most easily by a loop cholecystojejunostomy using an intraluminal circular stapler. While not as durable a biliary decompressive procedure as a hepatico-jejunostomy, it is much easier to construct technically. If the patient already has an endobiliary stent, there is less need for a formal operative biliary bypass. A gastroenterostomy to a loop of jejunum can be performed either anticolic or retrocolic using a linear cutting stapler or a endoluminal circular stapler passed proximally through the same enterotomy used for the cholecystojejunostomy.

## Laparoscopic Pancreatectomy

The first laparoscopic distal pancreatectomy was performed by Cuschieri in 1994, and, subsequently, the procedure has been further refined with newer techniques in regard to the preservation of the spleen and the management of the pancreatic distal remnant. Several large series have been reported with good success and results similar to those of open distal pancreatectomies. Although there are anecdotal reports of proximal pancreatectomies (pancreatoduodenectomies), the advantages claimed are not evident, the duration of the operative has been very long, and this approach remains unproven at this time.

*Indications*: At the moment, the primary indications for a laparoscopic pancreatectomy should be restricted to benign pathology and low-grade malignancies. The most frequent indications are insulinomas, serous and mucinous cystic neoplasms, neuroendocrine neoplasms, and chronic pancreatitis. Laparoscopic distal pancreatectomy for typical ductal cancer is usually less feasible, because these neoplasms are often diagnosed in advanced stages that may obviate a safe laparoscopic approach.

*Technique*: The patient is positioned on the operating table to allow a right lateral position with the left arm at an arch of 90° with the thorax. We utilize three 10 mm trocars and one of

5 mm in diamond-shaped disposition (umbilical, subxiphoid, left and right subcostal). We begin the dissection with the mobilization of the splenic flexure of the colon (Fig. 13.3a) to allow complete exposure of the lower pole of the spleen, the splenic hilum, and the tail of the pancreas (Fig. 13.3b).

With the harmonic scalpel, the gastrocolic ligament is transected exposing the anterior surface of the body and tail of the pancreas; initially we preserve the short gastric vessels. We begin the dissection of the pancreas by dividing the thin peritoneum that fixes the lower edge to retroperitoneum, from medial to lateral toward the splenic hilum, taking care not to injure the splenic vein that may adhere to the posterior aspect of the pancreas. Subsequently, we transect the peritoneum that covers the upper edge of the pancreas, where the splenic artery can usually be visualized.

Once the splenic vessels are located, a plane must be created between them and the pancreatic parenchyma proximal to the pancreatic pathology. This plane allows placement of the linear stapler to transect the neck of the pancreas (Fig. 13.3c).

If appropriate, attempts at splenic preservation can be carried out (benign disease or cystic neoplasms of low potential for invasive malignancy). By ventral and lateral retraction of the distal pancreas with forceps, the arterial and venous branches of the pancreatic vessels can be visualized and controlled with the use of harmonic scalpel or clips up to the hilum of the spleen (Fig. 13.3d).

Once the distal pancreatectomy is completed, the resected specimen is placed into a plastic bag and extracted through a slightly enlarged port site. Finally, a closed-suction drain is placed in the bed of the pancreatic resection and exteriorized through one of the 5 mm port sites.

## Laparoscopic Treatment of Insulinomas

As insulinomas are benign in more than 90% of patients, these are ideal neoplasms for enucleation laparoscopically if possible. The advantage of laparoscopy in the management of these neoplasms is based on the amplification of the field of vision afforded by laparoscopy as well as the minimal access approach for simple enucleation. The disadvantage of a laparoscopic approach is the inability to formally palpate the gland, an important step in the open surgery for the intraoperative localization; however, intraoperative localization can be aided by the use of intraoperative laparoscopy.

The preliminary results of laparoscopic enucleation of insulinomas seem to be favorable, provided the localization of the neoplasm is obtained preoperatively. The reported mortality and morbidity are 0% and 16%, respectively.

*Technique*: The patient is placed supine with the legs spread and the surgeon positioned between the patient's legs. Access involves four trocars: two of 10 mm (umbilical, right subcostal) and two of 5 mm (left subcostal and subxiphoid). We begin with the dissection very similar to that for a laparoscopic distal pancreatectomy by opening widely the gastrocolic ligament. In this manner, we obtain access to the lesser sac with the exposure of the body and tail of the pancreas. The head of the pancreas can be exposed by careful dissection of the hepatocolic connections and the gastrocolic ligament, with special care to control the right gastroepiploic vein to expose the head and neck of the pancreas where it joins with the superior mesenteric vein. Once the anterior face of the pancreas is exposed completely, inspection with laparoscopic ultrasonography is performed (Fig. 13.4). Once the location of the tumor is confirmed, then the type of resection will be decided, according to size, anatomic location, and the relationship between the neoplasm and the main pancreatic duct. If the tumor is superficial, it is amenable to a safe laparoscopic enucleation. If enucleation is not feasible, then a spleen-preserving distal pancreatectomy may be performed with splenic vessel preservation for insulinomas in the body or tail of the gland. Insulinomas in the head and uncinate process may be amenable to laparoscopic enucleation, but their exposure can be much more problematic laparoscopically.

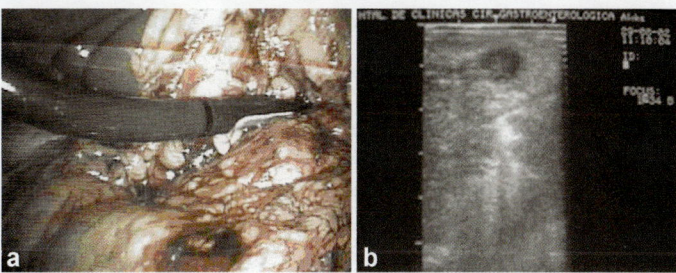

FIGURE 13.4. Intraoperative localization of an insulinoma with laparoscopic ultrasonography. (**a**) Laparoscopic ultrasonic transducer in contact with the anterior face of the pancreas. (**b**) Intraoperative ultrasonography of a 1 cm insulinoma adjacent to but not in contact with the pancreatic duct.

## Laparoscopic Drainage of Pancreatic Pseudocyst

Most patients with pancreatic pseudocysts are managed currently by endoscopic internal transgastric or transduodenal drainage. Combined laparo-endoscopic techniques have been described by placing transmural trocars into the stomach to allow better visualization and approach to transgastric internal drainage. This approach as well as laparoscopic anastomosis between the adjacent wall of the pseudocyst and the stomach using a linear cutting stapler have also been described, but again, offer little or no advantage to endoscopic drainage for pseudocysts adherent to the wall of the stomach.

In contrast, for pancreatic pseudocysts not amenable to endoscopic transgastric or trans-duodenal drainage, it is possible to perform a laparoscopic or laparoscopic-assisted internal drainage into the jejunum, usually a Roux limb. This technique can be performed infracolically when the pseudocyst protrudes through the mesocolon or antecolically after opening the gastrocolic ligament. The pseudocysto-jejunostomy can be stapled laparoscopically or hand-sewn.

# Laparoscopic Necrosectomy for Acute Necrotizing Pancreatitis

Laparoscopic and other minimal access approaches have been described for the operative management of infected pancreatic and peripancreatic necrosis. As the goal of a necrosectomy is to remove only the necrotic material, minimal access approaches seem ideally suited to this disease.

*Indications*: Because pancreatic necroses must partially liquify and separate from viable surrounding tissue to allow a safe, non-anatomic necrosectomy, a minimal access approach is most amenable in patients who are usually 3 or more weeks out after onset of the disease and who have relatively localized necrosis – usually in the lesser sac anterior to the body and neck of the gland. Necrosectomy is best indicated for infected necrosis or for patients with symptomatic, walled-off necrosis who are not getting better with conservative management.

*Technique*: In general, the minimal access approaches involve either a fully laparoscopic approach or a laparoscopic-assisted, minimal access, focused open approach. Access to the area of necrosis is usually obtained by a percutaneous drain placed under computed tomography guidance. The tract of this drain is then dilated gradually over a wire to allow an operating, perfused nephroscope to enter the area of necrosis. A necrosectomy can then be performed by placing laparoscopic forceps through the channel of the nephroscope. This technique uses both manual debridement and continuous irrigation to effect the necrosectomy and may require several sessions to complete the necrosectomy.

A related technique involves making a small incision subcostally in the flank or lateral abdominal wall, locating the drain, and following its entrance into the area of necrosis. Through this small incision, a 10 mm trocar and laparoscope can be inserted, and the necrosectomy monitored visually through the laparoscope. A finger, forceps can be placed alongside the laparoscope to effect the necrosectomy.

After both these techniques, a closed-system irrigation can be established to lavage the cavity continuously for several days to 2 weeks to maximize both the necrosectomy as well as drainage of the cavity should extravasation of pancreatic secretions occur. Results are similar to open necrosectomy but this technique avoids the morbidity of a major celiotomy. Patients for minimal access necrosectomy should, however, be selected carefully.

## Selected Readings

Brunt LM (2004) Laparoscopic partial gastrectomy. Oper Tech Gen Surg 6:29–41

Cuschieri A (2000) Minimal access surgery – laparoscopic gastric resection. Surg Clin N Am 80:1269–1284

Kitano S, Shiraishi N (2005) Minimally invasive surgery for gastric tumors. Surg Clin N Am 85:151–164

Mabrut J, Fernandez Cruz L, Azagra J, et al. (2005) Laparo-scopic pancreatic resection: results of a multicenter European study of 127 patients. Surgery 137:178–184

Minnard E, Conlon K, Hoos A, et al. (1998) Laparoscopic ultrasound enhances standard laparoscopy in the staging of pancreatic cancer. Ann Surg 228:182–187

Warshaw A, Gu Z, Wittemberg J, et al. (1990) Preoperative staging and assessment of resectability of pancreatic cancer. Arch Surg 125: 230–233

# Index